Armed and Dangerous

Armed and Dangerous

Fit, Firm and Ready to Fight

WENDY and BARB

KEY PORTER BOOKS

Canadian Cataloguing in Publication Data

Buckland, Wendy
    Armed and dangerous : fit, firm and ready to fight

ISBN 1-55013-798-0

1. Health.   2. Low-fat diet.   3. Low-fat diet - Recipes.
I. Nicoll, Barb   II. Title

RA776.B83   1996   613   C96-930892-2

The publisher gratefully acknowledges the assistance of the
Canada Council and the Ontario Arts Council.

Key Porter Books Limited
70 The Esplanade
Toronto, Ontario
Canada M5E 1R2

Design: Jean Lightfoot Peters and Leah Gryfe
Electronic Formatting: Heidi Palfrey

Printed and bound in Canada

96 97 98 99 6 5 4 3 2 1

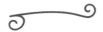

Contents

This book is dedicated to ...

★ my Mom, my greatest inspiration and role model;
★ my son, Lee, a great kid that I'm always proud of;
★ my family, the audience with loudest cheers of encouragement;
★ Bill, the love of my life;
★ Lori, my sister and best friend

W.B.

Brian
★ you always believed in me;
★ you always loved me;
★ without you there would be nothing!
Thank you.

Mom
★ what a special person you are;
★ always there for me and my family!
I love you.

Jake
★ my wonderful son;
★ I want to give you a beautiful life!

B.N.

Preface

One day, several months ago, I came upon an interesting sight in a local supermarket: a group of shoppers were studying, deciphering and assessing the nutritional information on food labels.

What's more, they were having fun! Led by two bubbly, enthusiastic women named Wendy Buckland and Barb Nicoll, the shoppers were discovering the disturbingly high levels of fat in many common foods, and discussing the effects on their weight and health.

Soon, Wendy and Barb had me sampling their products (their delicious no-fat bruschetta won me over immediately!).

Their timing couldn't be better. Medical evidence supports the need to make drastic cuts in the fat levels of North American diets. The proof is simply overwhelming, especially for the prevention of lifestyle-related conditions, such as heart disease and stroke—diseases that happen to be the leading cause of death in people over the age of forty.

To those of us in the medical profession, this may be old news. What's fresh and exciting is the way in which the message is being spread—with lots of laughter and anecdotes . . . and no lectures. We're all human, after all, and we would rather skip down the road of least resistance than scale a steep mountain of proof.

That's the appeal of Wendy and Barb's message. It includes:

★ delicious low-fat recipes;

★ activities that are fun to do;

★ a de-emphasis on calories and fad diets;

★ sensible advice about the foods we eat and the ingredients we use.

Your lifestyle is the only factor you can change in order to improve your overall health and life span. Wendy and Barb are to be congratulated for having delivered this very important message in an easy to understand, entertaining and down-to-earth style.

So, please—read on and enjoy *Armed and Dangerous*. I wish you success in the pursuit of your new and healthier lifestyle.

L. Bergin, MD
Cardiologist

An Assistant Professor, Department of Medicine, at the University of Western Ontario, Dr. Bergin has been certified in both Internal Medicine and Cardiology by the American Board of Internal Medicine and the Royal College of Physicians & Surgeons of Canada.

CHAPTER ONE

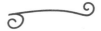

Who Needs More Pain?

It always begins with advice. Asking other people for advice about losing weight is an easy thing to do. Getting advice back is even easier. That's because most people approach the subject of losing weight and getting fit like they do politics: They always have an opinion, and if you don't like this week's opinion, come back for a new one next week.

Okay, we have our opinions too. But what you'll read in the following pages is different in a number of ways.

First, everything you read here is something we have lived through ourselves. We're not academics or scientists. We're two reasonable, ordinary people who found ways to lose weight and get fit because we were determined to.

Second, we're not so different from you. We don't relish the feeling of pain, hunger or guilt any more than you do. One of the dumbest bits of advice tossed around in recent years is "No pain, no gain." That's not a guideline for helping you feel better about the state of your body—it's a rallying cry for a society of masochists!

Third, we enjoy having fun. And we've tried to make this book fun to read and easy to follow.

Finally, beyond a certain age, staying slim and fit becomes something of a battle. Like all battles, the winners will be the ones with the best strategy, the most powerful weapons and the strongest morale.

That's our side. And we're looking for recruits.

The way we see it, everyone's life has enough pain as it is without adding more. We know—we've had our share, just like everyone else.

Every woman who has given birth, passed a kidney stone or recovered from major surgery has experienced all the physical pain she needs, thank you very much. And let's not get into the pain of falling in love with someone who has fallen out of love with you.

Feeling better about your body shouldn't have anything to do with feeling pain. In most cases, pushing your body beyond its limits is totally unnecessary, and in many cases it can be downright harmful. Pain is your body's way of saying "Stop whatever you're doing or I'll slip a disk! Or tear a ligament! Or develop arthritic joints!" Ignore your body's warnings and you'll pay for it, either now or later—because your body never forgets and rarely forgives.

In this case, "pain" doesn't mean just the agony of physical exertion or emotional trauma. If the thrill of biting into a hot french fry or a cheeseburger-with-the-works borders on orgasmic for you, and always has, it hurts to hear someone declare: "Thou shall not consume another fry, burger or hot dog!" Denial is painful in its own way too. Life is to be enjoyed, and you can enjoy being healthy and still enjoy a sinful treat now and then.

We know. We've done it, and we continue to do it. And we overcame some good-sized barriers to do it.

But that's enough talk about that. From now on there'll be no talk of suffering pain, no preaching about committing sins and, most of all, no heavy doses of guilt.

You don't need them in your life. And we don't need them to make our point. Because everything you need to become the person you want to be already exists in three places:

★ at your supermarket;

★ in your home;

★ between your ears;

We're all stronger than we think we are.

Most of us underestimate our own talents. We're usually too modest about our own capabilities, both mental and physical. In fact, if our ancestors a hundred thousand years ago had said, "Heck, I'll never be able to do that!," we'd still be living in trees, eating bananas (Try that during a Saskatoon winter!) and dodging other animals that love us, not for our minds, but for our bodies—as dinner.

It's a cruel fact of life, but it's still true: It takes adversity to reveal just how strong we are and how many things we're capable of doing well.

That's why the most successful business people often begin life in poverty and hunger. (And why the spoiled children of rich parents often mature into addle-headed adults who tear down everything their parents have accomplished.)

A Word from Wendy:

Now and then, one of us will step forward, so to speak, and talk "one-on-one" to you. I'm first.

Many parts of my life were painful and depressing. Big deal, right? So whose life isn't from time to time?   But every now and then it hits me: If I hadn't had juvenile rheumatoid arthritis and bone reconstruction and a kidney removed and a bunch of other heartbreak, I would have been more like some of the women I grew up with—the ones who dated the good-looking boys, married the successful men and lived in the perfect suburban houses.

Would I have been happier? Who knows? But I know this:

I wouldn't be as strong as I am now. Not just physically, but mentally and emotionally.

You've heard it all before, but it's true: Perfect human bodies exist only in the minds of air-brush artists at *Playboy*.

So here's my point:

Face your weaknesses (or at least the ones that affect your

looks ands health). Stare them right in the eye. Determine to overcome just them, and you'll achieve much more than you planned on.

Talk to you later....

We're all strong in different places. Where's yours?

Anybody remember *Butch Cassidy and the Sundance Kid*? If you're a woman over forty, you must recall that movie. No woman who saw it can forget the sight of a young Paul Newman and a young Robert Redford wearing cowboy clothes and acting like decent men in the Old West.

The most memorable scene in the movie for many people occurs about halfway through. Newman and Redford (or "Butch" and "Sundance," if you want to get familiar) have robbed trains, dispatched bullies, climbed mountains and ridden their horses into a lather—real macho stuff that makes Stallone's Rambo look like a wanna-be grease monkey. But the posse's after them, and eventually they find themselves trapped at the edge of a steep canyon.

Butch suggests they dive into the river to escape certain death or capture by the posse. The very thought makes Sundance look as though he's just been asked about having sexual relations with his horse. He's more than frightened and embarrassed—he's *humiliated*. In fact, he's so ashamed, Butch almost has to pry the reason from him:

Sundance can't swim.

It's a great comic moment because it contrasts with the otherwise heroic qualities of the man—he can do so many things that others won't even attempt, but *he never learned to swim*.

It's also funny because it taps into an emotion all of us have felt at some time in our lives (and many feel every day): The awareness that we don't possess certain abilities other people take for granted. And that's humiliating.

If you're reading this book, one of those strengths you lack— or *think* you lack—is the ability to shape both your body and your life until they match your image. This is no trivial matter. To coin a phrase, it's easy to say "It's easy," but for many people things are never that simple.

If the Robert Redford character could accomplish everything else he achieved in *Butch Cassidy and the Sundance Kid*, he could have learned to swim as well. All he needed was a helping hand and a few basic facts.

So, in moments of self-doubt, just picture yourself teaching a young Robert Redford to swim. (We will pause here, if necessary, to permit our female readers to stare off into space and smile quietly to themselves.)

How to measure and apply the strength within you.

You don't need a pencil for this, but it helps. (And if you use a pencil, be sure not to lend this book to a friend. Or your spouse. Or your mother. Not to mention any bitchy siblings.)

Besides, writing things down tends to make them real. So, even though you may be able to answer these questions in your head, the act of writing changes them from thoughts and wishes to facts.

It's all very simple:

My Three Biggest Weaknesses	My Three Biggest Strengths
1. _____	1. _____
2. _____	2. _____
3. _____	3. _____

Let yourself go on this one. If you determine that your biggest weakness is that you can't pass a hamburger stand without wanting to sell your (pick one) ❑ Soul; ❑ Body; ❑ First-born Kid; ❑ Car for a greasy cheeseburger you can call your own, admit it. Be honest to the point of brutality: *"I have no self-control over the fat I put into my body!!!!"* If your weakness is the opposite sex, write it down. Talk to yourself honestly about the things you encounter each day that defeat you, one way or another.

It doesn't matter what you write on those three lines— although we'll bet at least one of them has something to do with what you eat and how you look. What matters is proving and admitting one thing to yourself:

You are human. You are imperfect. You have weaknesses. And, because of these qualities, you are capable of being exploited. By whom? How long a list do you want? By lovers and food companies, lawyers and sales clerks, your kids and your mother, your cat and your dog, and on and on. Not all the exploitation is bad or painful. The sales clerk who tells you how great you look in that new skirt is exploiting you to make a sale, but she's also making you feel good. If that's what you need and you can afford it, go ahead.

The art of being wise is the art of knowing what to overlook.

WILLIAM JAMES

During the 1980s, we heard a lot about "arming the consumer"—providing shoppers with the facts they need to spend their money wisely and receive full value for it. Some major companies went along with the idea reluctantly. General Motors, for example, had failed for years to tell buyers of expensive Oldsmobiles and Buicks that the engine in their car may be identical to the engines in Chevrolets costing thousands of dollars less. A lot of people were upset by the news, and now GM and all the other car companies put it in writing: Here's what you get, and here's what it means.

Consumers became armed with information about the material in their clothes as well. Can I wash it? Can I bleach it? Does it need dry-cleaning? North American industry has armed consumers since the 1970s, providing us with the ammunition we need to take charge of the things we buy.

But if we have the weapons and refuse to use them, whose fault is that? Consider the tobacco industry. Smokers get dumped on enough as it is, and even the tobacco hucksters are finally admitting that nicotine is a narcotic. But if somebody sold you a sweater with a label that said: *Notice: Wearing this garment has been proven to cause cancer*, how often would you put the darn thing on? If you're a smoker and ignore the warnings on the cigarette packages, you're armed but you've already surrendered.

So whether you're buying a Buick or a brassiere, you're armed with information these days, and nobody can say you weren't warned.

Why is it that we will spend more time examining the washing instructions of something we'll wear *on* our bodies than we spend examining the ingredients of things we'll put *in* our bodies? Does that make any sense? Unless you or a member of your family has a serious allergy problem, the chances are you don't examine the ingredients of the food you eat as carefully as you should.

Food companies, to one extent or another, are providing you with the ammunition you need to make better decisions for your health. This book will arm you with the facts to fire back.

Okay, you've written your three biggest weaknesses in the left column. Now look at the right column. What are your strengths? And don't be modest here! If you're one heck of a cook, or someone with real empathy around children and old folks, put it down. Brag a little. Balance that other column, and even tip it in your favor somewhat. Include certain strengths or talents even if you're the only one who's impressed by them. (After yourself, who else do you need to impress anyway?)

If your main talent is that you can still name every tune on the Beatles' *Sgt. Pepper* album and you're proud of it, good for you. If you can be so concerned about your own inner peace that you devote at least half an hour every day to spending time alone, that's a terrific strength—take pride in it! If you're loyal to your friends no matter what, boast about it to yourself.

Just remember this: *Every strength leads to a talent.* And every talent can be used to change your life according to your needs and your values—no one else's. Talent is ammunition to use when arming yourself against pain, distress and failure. It all begins by acknowledging the talent you have and aiming it in the right direction. Here are a few examples of things you might have listed as strengths, and how they can help make you *Armed and Dangerous* when it comes to eating right, feeling better and staying fit:

★ *I'm a good parent.* Congratulations—in case you've never thought about it, you're successful at the most challenging and difficult job in the world. (And you usually get such poor on-the-job training too!) Good parents are caregivers, moral guideposts, and sources of comfort and support. If you can provide those things for your kids, you can provide them for yourself.

★ *I'm financially responsible.* Another tough job, especially these days. It takes knowledge, self-control and the ability to keep your eye on a target to avoid slipping into serious debt. (A little good luck doesn't hurt either.) You're already armed. All you need now is another target.

★ *I dress well.* That's not a frivolous ability. It usually means good self-assessment, an appreciation for color and form, and at least a reasonable concern about your physical appearance. Getting the picture here?

★ *I have attractive eyes*—or good hair, decent cheekbones, shapely legs, whatever. Take your best feature, the one you don't have to work at, and start adding to it. It's part of your body, after all, and it's your body—the entire package—that we're starting with here. Your self-esteem will follow—not because the rest of the world suddenly discovers how good you look, but because you know who was responsible for making the change.

★ *I have many friends.* They're an invaluable asset. Use them.

★ *I'm reasonably intelligent.* Of course you are. You bought this book, didn't you?

Now circle one of the strengths on your list. Use a red pencil or marker if you like. Put a check mark at the top of page 13. Remember the talent you have that's responsible for that strength. Then, anytime, anywhere, when reading this book or when you're having doubts about your ability to achieve your goal in weight and fitness, come back to the list.

It's your source of ammunition. It's what keeps you armed against all the people and things out there that prevent you from doing what you and your body know must be done.

You're on your way to becoming dangerous.

A Note from Barb:

After the birth of my beautiful boy, Jake, something happened to my body . . . and then to my self. It's hardly unique to new mothers, but that makes it all the more important.

In a word, I expanded. I grew HUGE! Me, the slim kid on the block, grew almost as big as the block itself. I soon weighed 190 pounds and I was so embarrassed—not just at my weight, but at whatever weakness was causing me to mushroom—that I became a short-term hermit, staying inside so the rest of the world wouldn't catch a glimpse of me. Once inside, of course, I discovered all kinds of things to do. Like nibble on food and watch TV. And yes, I saw women on some of the TV shows saying the same kinds of things I'm saying now, about how they once had a weight problem too. Mind you, a lot of them solved it by investing in some kind of device that looked like a cross between a mountain bike and a freight elevator, which they bought with twenty-four easy monthly payments, but that's another story . . .

Anyway, it all seemed so unfair! Here I had this beautiful baby boy, on the one hand, and I was paying for it with a body shape I didn't want, on the other hand.

So I was in a spiral, and the only direction was down. Don't look good? Stay home. Staying home? Let's eat! Eating too much of the wrong things? You don't look good. Don't look good? Stay home!

I'd heard all the horror stories about trying to lose weight by reducing calories, and I didn't want more disappointment. Working with one of those twenty-four-easy-payment torture machines didn't seem like the best solution either. I needed something that would be long-term, easy to manage, and nutritionally sound. After all, this was my body we're talking about. There may have been more of it than I wanted at the time, but it was still mine, and I wasn't going to abuse it.

Then I thought about cruise control. You know, that little button on the dashboard of a lot of cars these days? You set it once at the speed you want, and the car maintains it. At first, I thought it was just another dumb guy-thing gimmick. You take your foot off the gas and the car obediently keeps going, following your every command. But then somebody pointed out the real advantage of cruise control:

It keeps you from getting speeding tickets.

Most people who get speeding tickets on the highway can't believe they're going as fast as the cop says they are. On an open highway on a clear dry day, it's easy for your speed to creep up without your knowing it—until the flashing red light appears in the window and the cop shows you the radar reading that says you were clipping along at 80 mph (130 kph). Cruise control wouldn't let you do it. All you have to do is set the limit, and everything else takes care of itself. (You still have to steer the car, but you get the idea....)

If there was a form of cruise control for eating—where all you had to do was set a mark and eat anything under that level—maybe we wouldn't get pulled over, so to speak. Maybe we could just relax, enjoy life, and watch the scenery go by.

That's what Wendy taught me, and it's the basic reason why I leap around the stage at our seminars, proudly wear a size 8, and am so pleased when other women approach me and say "Boy, I wish I looked like you!"

Cruise control. Think about it.

Let's stop blaming the victims.

A lot of us are concerned about laws that seem to blame the victim. It started with sexual-assault cases. For years, society believed that women who dressed a certain way or went to certain places were "asking for it." When whatever "it" was happened, we tended to blame the person it happened to. And that's wrong. A woman who walks into a bar alone at night wearing a tight dress may be guilty of bad judgment, or even sheer stupidity, but she's not guilty of inviting gang rape, if that's what happens. It's the other people who are guilty—the ones who saw her as a potential victim in the first place, and took advantage of the situation.

We're not riding a feminist horse here. We both like men; we think most of them are neat, a few of them are wonderful, a bunch of them are sewer rats and, like it or not, they're all here to stay. We're also mothers of sons whom we love, and some day they're going to join that mix of adult humanity on the other side of the gender fence.

But blaming the victim is wrong, whether we're talking sexual harassment or an inability to have the kind of body a person wants to have. We're not talking self-control. We're talking about a kind of passive victimization—in this instance, against both men *and* women.

For too long, all of us have allowed ourselves to become nutrition victims. Walking into a supermarket without being aware of the effects that some food products can have on our bodies is like walking into a Hell's Angels party and thinking it's a Rotary Club meeting. We believe what the package label tells us. We're aware of basic nutrition rules and we're especially responsive to friendly introductions and sincere smiles. Frankly, it reminds us of a singles bar. On the supermarket shelves, the smiles and introductions translate into pick-up lines:

> *Calorie-Reduced!*
> *Low Fat!*
> *No Cholesterol!*
> *Diet Formula!*
> *Reduced Fat!*

Hey, if you've had trouble squeezing into your slacks that morning, those kinds of words go straight to your heart, don't they? It's only afterwards that you learn the real truth of the matter—and then it's too late.

The time to take control of your health, your body and your life is when you make those supermarket purchases, not on the basis of sexy packaging and whatever messages your taste buds are sending you, but on the information tucked away on the back—especially items like fat content. That's the "cruise control" idea that Barb talked about. If you control your fat intake by keeping it below a certain level—think of it as your body's "speed limit"—you'll never get caught feeding more fat calories into your body than it can handle.

Heroism, the Sherpa mountaineers say, is endurance for one moment more.

GEORGE KENNAN

The good news is that food companies are finally putting all this information on their packages—the equivalent of clothing manufacturers telling you whether you can bleach their garment; if you should dry clean it; and just how much polyester, cotton or whatever they've used to make the thing.

The bad news is that few of us are reading, calculating, understanding and applying all this important data.

Oh yeah, more good news:

Years ago, talking about things like low-fat content usually meant kissing your appetite good-bye, because much of the flavor and enjoyment of food was tied directly to fat content. Well, things have changed. We know a fast-food chain that sells an all-vegetable burger containing almost zero fat so toothsome that we defy you—*defy you*—to recognize that it contains not one gram of dead cow.

Another Note from Wendy:

Unfortunately, we've all gone through the disappointment of sampling foods with reduced calories only to find we miss the taste associated with "the real thing." Well, things have changed. If we can build a computer that talks to us and does our tax return, we can certainly create a food that cuts fat substantially without changing things like taste and texture very much. And we can. We proved it, Barb and I.

Pardon the commercial message here, but when Barb and I launched our company, we wanted to prove that eliminating excess fat didn't have to make a noticeable difference in taste and texture. So we began by developing recipes for three products: bruschetta, hummus and baba-ghanouj, each with full flavor but less fat.

Bruschetta was relatively easy; ours has 0 percent fat. Zilch, nada, none at all. Some prepackaged products use olive oil but, by adjusting other ingredients, you can avoid the oil content and never miss it.

Hummus, made with chick-peas and tahini butter (from sesame seeds), typically has about 45 percent fat content in the calories.[1] That's too high; we reduced ours to less than 30 percent, or just two-thirds of that.

Baba-ghanouj was a bigger challenge. A combination of eggplant, oil, garlic and spices, it's the kind of dip and spread whose flavor will curl the toes of your taste buds. Normally, about 75 percent of its calorie content is derived from fat. We set ourselves a limit of 20 percent fat content (as measured against total calories—we'll explain the calculation details later, and it's pretty simple to work out). And we did it. We have a product that will keep your bridge club/poker night/cocktail party set raving, and all of them will be consuming about a third as much fat as normal, without knowing it.

Once we perfected the recipe, we found a small, high-quality food company to manufacture all three products for us and persuaded some major grocery-store chains to sell it.

This sounds like a sales pitch, and in a way it is. But, more important, it's here as proof of the fact that, after putting men on the moon and women in executive suites (not enough of either you might say, but that's another story...), modern society has found a way to honestly cut fat content without affecting flavor. Hey, it's a start!

By the way, the villains in this book aren't food companies or supermarkets. They exist to provide us what we ask for, and who can fault them for that? The villain is fat. Like all villains, fat has its good and bad side. Unfortunately, the bad side is the one that causes all the pain and suffering.

So let's get it out front: Our bodies need fat—*some* fat. It's as essential to our all-round health as vitamins, minerals, roughage and other ingredients. We're not out to *eliminate* fat from our food; we're out to *control* it, because almost all of us are eating far more fat in our food than we should. How much more? It varies, but some nutritionists claim *five times as much as we need, or more.*

Fat alone isn't a bad thing. The problem is, we're all eating far too much of a not-so-bad thing. In the case of fat, this suddenly becomes disastrous.

---

[1] For our calorie-content ratings, we used Karen Bellerson's *The Complete and Up-to-Date Fat Book*, (Garden City Park, NY: Avery, 1993).

It's not a fad and it's not fashion—it's your life we're talking about here!

Is low-fat just another one of those talk-show topics that everyone natters about for half an hour before moving on to more serious matters—like where *was* O.J. that night?

Take this to the bank: *Low-fat is not a fad.* It's a legitimate response from a society that is finally paying close attention to the effects of excess fat on their health, their lifestyle, their well-being and their time on this planet. It is also, in our opinion, a natural extension of our changed attitudes toward smoking.

Our grandchildren will find it amusing, appalling or both that people felt free to light up a cigarette in almost any public location they chose and to spew their smoke into the air. Smoking was once considered a fashionable pastime. Now, in virtually every public place, it's seen as boorish behavior. More important, it took barely a decade for cigarettes to change from an attractive accessory to a barely tolerable bizarre habit.

True, the feeling isn't universal—yet. Too many people continue

Frequency of a heart attack in the United States:

1 every 25 seconds[2]

Frequency of death from a heart attack in the United States:

1 every 45 seconds[3]

---

[2]T. Gordon, "Premature Mortality from Coronary Heart Disease: The Framingham Study," *Journal of the American Medical Association,* 215 (1971), 1617; C. Baintin, "Deaths from Coronary Heart Disease," *New England Journal of Medicine*, 268 (1963), 569; W. Kannel, "Incidence and Prognosis of Unrecognized Myocardial Infarction—An Update on the Framingham Study," *New England Journal of Medicine*, 311 (1984), 1144.

[3]Ibid.

to smoke, and too many of them are young people who do it as much as a gesture of rebellion as a pleasurable diversion. *But the norm has changed*—smokers have changed from the normal majority (watched any 1950s movies lately?) to a barely endured minority.

Our approach to excess fat is changing the same way, and heading for the same goal. It's not a fad. It's a concept that runs far deeper than all that hype about oat bran, calcium and vitamin C. That kind of stuff is window-dressing when it comes to nutrition; fat is basic to everything we consume.

The key difference between tobacco and fat is that we all need fat. Nothing—absolutely nothing—in our bodies needs nicotine to function well.

Another Word from Barb:

Notice that we haven't used the "D" word here. You know, that four-letter word that follows terms like "Scarsdale" and "Grapefruit"? We'll talk about it more in the next chapter, but for now we want to focus totally on fat.

The reason? To most people, the "D" word means failure. We've heard that as many as 98 percent of people who consider the "D" word as a solution to weight and health problems fail to reach their goal and remain there. That's only a 2 percent success rate! If you succeeded at only 2 percent of everything you did, wouldn't you start questioning either (a) what you're doing, or (b) your ability to do it right? Most people would assume (b)—they're just not equipped to do something as simple as control their food intake. The result is a loss of self-esteem and a prevailing "What's the use?" attitude.

So we'll deal with the "D" word briefly—*very briefly*—in the next chapter. Then we'll get on with the things you can do that will totally reverse the situation.

Fat isn't a total villain. The problem begins, not by eating any fat, but from eating too much of the stuff—more than we can either use or discard. So it hangs around our bodies like an unwanted house guest, taking up room, getting in the way and leaving its dirty laundry on the floor.

Here's what the proper amount of fat can do for us that's good:

★ Fat helps us fight disease. It is used by our bodies to create antibodies that fight viruses and bacteria.

★ Fat helps carry certain fat-soluble vitamins to the various places in our bodies where they can be used.

★ Fat makes good cushions (no surprise there, right?). Organs such as our kidneys, heart and liver are all surrounded by small fat deposits.

★ Fat helps our digestion, slowing down the stomach's production of hydrochloric acid.

So fat isn't all bad. In fact, it's a bit like the family cat or dog. When it's small and placid, a little fat is nice to have around. It makes you comfortable and provides some pleasure. But that works only if the fat doesn't get too big. Would you really want to share your home life with a three-hundred-pound tabby cat? Not likely. In fact, you wouldn't have any life to share at all, once your three-hundred-pound puss started looking at you as if you were a walking can of tuna.

That's what fat's like. Keep it down to size and it's good company. Let it get out of control, and it'll kill you. Count on it.

It may be tempting to say, "Hey, fat's good for me after all!" and reach for a bag of potato chips and a quart of sour-cream dip. Please don't. Here's why:

Our bodies are smart. Smarter than the other parts of us, in some ways. Since our bodies need a certain amount of fat, they have learned how to produce it from non-fatty parts of our food. The fats our bodies produce are called *non-essential fatty acids*, and if we remain reasonably healthy, we make all that we need without any outside help, thank you very much.

Unfortunately, our bodies aren't perfect. (Wow, there's an eye-opening statement, right?) Some kinds of fat our bodies need to stay healthy cannot be homemade, so to speak. They must be imported in our food. These are known as *essential fatty acids*, and they promote normal growth, healthy skin and blood systems, and keep our metabolism running smoothly.

But, guess what? On average, we need one tablespoon (15 mL) of fat—those essential fatty acids—per day. And it needn't be animal fat, either; we do very well with fatty acids from vegetable fats such as canola oil, olive oil, safflower oil and others.

Amount of food protein obtained from vegetable sources in 1900:

70 percent

Amount of food protein obtained from vegetable sources in 1990:

30 percent[4]

One of the few times we'll talk like nutritional experts— please bear with us.

The next few paragraphs are going to sound a little like a textbook. Sorry about that, but it's important to define terms such as "saturated fat," "polyunsaturated fat," "monounsaturated fat" and "cholesterol." Why? Because all four terms show up on food labels at your supermarket, and many people are confused about their importance.

Let's start with the real villain in the story: saturated fat. It's the killer.

Saturated fats are almost always solid at room temperature. Think of any fatty food that is both solid and greasy, and you have

---

[4]Michael Chatterson and Linda Chatterson, *The Final Diet* (Salt Lake City: Northwest Publishing, 1994).

yourself a chunk of saturated fat. These include animal-derived products such as butter and cheese, and fats from tropical oils such as coconut and palm oil. You like chocolate? Well, the basis of all chocolate is cocoa butter, and cocoa butter is 100 percent saturated fat.

These are the fats to avoid—or at least reduce—at all costs. So, be suspicious and selective when it comes to choosing any foods based on animals, dairy products or tropical oils.

Another Word from Wendy

I almost died when I heard the bad news about chocolate. It's one of the great joys of life to me! Did I have to make a decision between eating low-fat and eating chocolate?

The answer was "Not really." If I could find some recipes that satisfied my craving for chocolate without including saturated fats, I could have the best of both worlds.

The idea was simple and difficult at the same time.

Simple idea: Keep the chocolate flavor while eliminating the fat. Difficult challenge: Doing it.

The point is that solutions do exist, if you spend a little time and effort to find them. And we did. Now it's up to you to sample and enjoy them!

Polyunsaturated fats are liquid at room temperature. You won't find these fats in animals, but you will find them in some fish. They're most commonly produced by plants as oils in nuts, seeds and soybeans. The presence of polyunsaturated fats in foods—especially cooking and salad oils—is usually trumpeted on the labels by the food manufacturers as though it's reason enough to buy the stuff. You know, the kids' cereal says *"Free Toy!"* and the salad dressings say *"Polyunsaturated Fat!"*

Polyunsaturated fats tend to reduce blood cholesterol, which makes them good for your body in moderate quantities. But they're still *fat*, which makes them unwelcome in large quantities.

Conditions that can be prevented or improved through avoidance of animal-based fat:[5]

Arthritis	*Asthma*
Breast Cancer	*Colon Cancer*
Constipation	*Diabetes*
Diverticulosis	*Gallstones*
Heart Disease	*Hypertension*
Hypoglycemia	*Kidney Disease*
Osteoporosis	*Prostate Cancer*
Stroke	

Monounsaturated fats are the almost-good-guys in the fat camp. They help reduce blood cholesterol just like their polyunsaturated siblings do, but they don't have some of the negative side effects of the poly group. So they're not so bad. *But they're still fat!* You'll find monounsaturated fats in nuts, chicken, oatmeal, avocados, ocean perch and other sources.

And now a word about (ugh!) hydrogenation.

So you have a batch of polyunsaturated and monounsaturated fats, ready to be enjoyed *in small quantities* by all of us health-conscious consumers. As long as you need a little fat, you can stick to these unsaturated guys and feel better, right?

Then someone comes along and hydrogenates those unsaturated fats. And guess what?

They take away the "un" from the word. Now you've got yourself nothing but trans-fatty acid, which behaves just like

---

[5]John McDougall, MD, *McDougall's Medicine: A Challenging Second Opinion* (Clinton, NJ: New Win, 1985); John McDougall and Mary A. McDougall, *The McDougall Plan* (Piscataway, NJ: New Century, 1983); John Robbins, *Diet for a New America* (Walpole, NH: Stillpoint, 1987).

saturated fats, those cholesterol-building, artery-clogging, life-shortening products that we've all been trying to avoid. Hydrogenation is a fairly simple process. Just add a bunch of hydrogen to the oil and you have solid saturated fats. That's hydrogenation. And it's bad news for your body.

Food processors use hydrogenated oils because they extend the life of baked goods, non-dairy creamers, whipped toppings and butter. It makes great sense from an economic and production standpoint. It makes little sense from a nutritional point of view. We need less fat and less hydrogen in the fat we consume.

The two most common elements in the universe are hydrogen and stupidity.
JOHN LAWRENCE REYNOLDS

Meanwhile, back in the arteries . . .

Cholesterol is the misunderstood child of the fat family. For one thing, it's ugly: white, waxy and fatty. And it has such unattractive origins: Most of the cholesterol we ingest comes from organ meats such as kidney, liver and, um, brains (also from shrimps, scallops and other animal sources).

Plants, by the way, cannot produce cholesterol. Eat all the vegetables you want, and you won't be putting any outside cholesterol into your system.

Cholesterol can get out of control, too, and then it becomes a hoodlum. Its most dangerous prank is clogging up our arteries, preventing the passage of blood and leading to high blood pressure, strokes and heart attacks.

The bright side of cholesterol? We need it. Cholesterol is the raw material for cell membranes. It also is used to manufacture bile acids, which aid digestion, and to produce major hormones such as estrogen, progesterone and testosterone.

From reasonably healthy meals, our bodies are pretty good at manufacturing all the cholesterol they need. Where? In our livers.

Now here's where it gets tricky, and if you want to skip to the end of this passage you won't miss much. But we think it's kind of interesting because it introduces a unique value of exercise and explains the way your body works, which is very important. The more you know about the way your body works, the better you can take care of it. Would you trust your car to a mechanic who never learned how to drive?

So our livers are sitting there, churning out cholesterol, to be used in building cell membranes and producing fun things such as estrogen, progesterone and testosterone. Question: How do you get the cholesterol to the places where it's needed? Answer: Carry it on the backs of things called "low-density lipoproteins," or LDLs. But these same LDLs, causing a traffic jam in our arteries, are the ones that lead to strokes, high blood pressure and all those other nasties. So a high level of LDLs is not good. Fortunately, the LDL level in your blood can be controlled by the kinds of food you eat, and by simple exercise.

Our bodies, recognizing that too much LDL is not a good thing, cleverly balance things by producing "high-density lipoproteins," or HDLs. The sole purpose of HDLs is to scour your body for excess cholesterol and carry it back to your liver, where a lot of it began in the first place. The liver sorts through all this unwanted cholesterol and discards the excess stuff from the body through the intestines.

To wrap things up:

High levels of low-density lipoproteins are not good, and are usually the result of eating too much of the wrong foods.

Low levels of high-density lipoproteins are not good either, and may be the result of not getting enough exercise.

Where do calories fit in?
It depends on what kind of calories you're trying to fit.

Long ago and far away, people learned to cut calories when trying to lose weight. The reasoning was simple: Calories provide energy, and excess calories are converted to something our bodies can store for future energy needs (read: *Fat*). Reduce your calorie intake and grow slim, right?

Well, life isn't as simple as that. (Life is *never* as simple as that.)

When measured by weight, carbohydrates and protein contain fewer calories per gram than fat—fewer than half as many, in fact. *Every gram of fat you eat provides your body with nine calories of energy; every gram of protein and carbohydrate brings just four calories with it.* This difference becomes very important when setting your "cruise control" to lose weight.

Also, the difference becomes even more critical when your body has to deal with all those calories from proteins and carbohydrates versus the same number of calories from fat. The fatty foods we eat are very similar to the fat in our bodies. When we digest these foods, the fats are separated and stockpiled in our bodies without much effort.

But the excess calories in proteins and carbohydrates must be processed by our bodies before they can be stored. Processing takes energy . . . and energy burns calories. By burning calories to convert them to fat, we actually reduce the impact of calories from protein and carbohydrates. Nutritionists tell us that we burn only 3 percent of the calories in fat to store it in our bodies for future use, but we burn 25 percent of the calories in proteins and carbohydrates to convert them to body fat.

As a result, that 9-to-4 ratio of calories in fat versus calories in equal weights of protein and carbohydrates translates to something closer to 9-to-3. Putting it another way, *the impact of calories from fat is three times as high as the impact of calories from proteins and carbohydrates, on a gram-for-gram basis.*

Barb's Turn:

This was a real eye-opener to me. Like most of you, I'd been raised to believe that a calorie is a calorie—they all wind up in the same place, which tends to be my hips. But a calorie from fat is much worse than a calorie from anywhere else, because it's just what is says it is—*fat*.

Think of tomatoes. If you bring home a case of canned tomatoes, all you have to do is stack them in your pantry and Presto! You've got a long-term supply of tomatoes taking up space.

But if you purchase a bushel of fresh tomatoes instead of the canned versions it becomes a different story. You have to skin them, place them in sterilized containers, seal the containers one by one, and do all the other processing chores necessary before shelving them. That's hard work, and you'd burn energy doing it.

Now think of the tomatoes as fat. Would you rather slap almost 100 percent of it on your hips, thighs, stomach and assorted other places? Or would you rather reduce it by at least 25 percent first? That's why it's just as important to recognize the source of calories as it is to measure their quantity.

So here's the picture: You want to lose weight. You've probably tried and failed in the past. So what? About 98 percent of people do, remember? Don't be so hard on yourself. You didn't fail at all. You just proved that you're human (there was any doubt?), and humans tend to avoid pain. Eliminating pleasure is a form of pain. Exercising beyond your needs is a form of pain. Denial is a form of pain. Beating yourself up mentally because you don't look like Cindy Crawford or Princess Di (or Mel Gibson or Hugh Grant, if you prefer) is a form of pain.

Arm yourself with knowledge to understand what your body needs and how to meet its needs without creating any of the pain described above. You'll soon start to see a change. Then you'll begin *feeling* a change. You'll feel successful (because you haven't "failed"). You'll feel confident (because nobody is putting one over on you about calories and fat content). You'll feel healthier, livelier and (wait for it) sexier.

Conscience is the inner voice that warns us somebody may be looking.

H. L. MENCKEN

We're not advocating that you become fashion-model thin. Not in the least. If you reduce your weight from 200 pounds to 150 pounds and decide to remain at that level, you still may be carrying more weight around than you ideally need, depending on your height. But hey—you're also that much healthier and happier too.

Kids, don't try this at home

If you have young children at home, don't include them in your low-fat diet without close consultation with your pediatrician.

To help their bodies develop normally, young children need higher levels of fat in their diet than adults do. If you feel your child has a weight problem, deal with it separately from your own by following a physician's guidance.

Besides, the less fat you carry, the better armed you are against things that can kill you—things like heart disease, cancer and stroke. All three are encouraged and even stimulated by excess fat in your body.

And all three are the leading causes of death among North Americans.

Check off these facts if you agree with them:

- ❑ Becoming slimmer and healthier doesn't have to be painful.
- ❑ I have weaknesses. So what? I also have strengths.
- ❑ If Butch Cassidy can admit his weaknesses, so can I.
- ❑ People are out to exploit me in nice and less-than-nice ways. It's up to me to arm myself to decide how, where and when I accept being exploited.
- ❑ Fat isn't all bad. But all-fat foods are *really* bad.
- ❑ If I can (a) find the right "speed" for my fat intake level and (b) "set" it in the foods I consume, I can relax and enjoy my meals without guilt.
- ❑ It helps to know about good cholesterol, bad cholesterol, and the difference between saturated and unsaturated fats, but it's not necessary.
- ❑ Hydrogenated foods are like unsafe sex.
- ❑ I can set a realistic weight goal, and relax when I reach it.

If you don't agree with a statement above, write your reasons here:

_____

_____

_____

_____

_____

_____

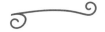

CHAPTER TWO

Why Are the Words "Diet" and "Common Sense" So Often Mutually Exclusive?

Here's where we finally mention the "D" word, as in "Scarsdale," "Grapefruit," "Eat-All-You-Want" and "Sorry-I'm-on-a."

Forget them all. The odds are about 50-to-1 against success in maintaining the new weight level you manage to reach. This includes programs set up by people who take your money so they can talk you into eating exclusively the foods they process—which means they take your money a second time.

We're not suggesting there is anything illegal, immoral, or even defective about most of these programs. We even believe the people behind them are well meaning. Just like the folks who make deep-fried potato chips, chocolate truffles and thick creamy Caesar salad dressing. The problem with diets is that *they succeed only if they change you from who you are into the person who created the diet wants you to be.*

Let's pause while you read the sentence again.

Look, you've spent two, three or four decades (or more) becoming a unique individual. You're probably not the person you originally set out to be (who is?), but in all the world, in all the universe, there is no one else who looks, thinks and acts exactly the way you do. It's a pleasant thought, and one we should all dwell on now and then.

But along comes someone who says "Eat this, don't eat that. Do this, don't do that. Be this person, don't be that person."

It's a seductive appeal, no question about it. Who doesn't want to be someone else now and then, for one reason or another? The trouble is, *it's impossible to transform yourself into someone else*, either physically or mentally. If you try, you're asking either for failure, which is what you'll almost certainly get; or dissatisfaction, because even if you succeed, you're now somebody else and whatever happened to *you*?

A Note from Wendy:

Barb and I come from very different backgrounds, and there is a fifteen-year difference in our ages. We don't agree on everything (sometimes we don't agree on *anything*!), including food, music, movies and fashion. When we conduct our seminars, we're very different people on stage, and we enjoy the difference. We agree on facts, however, and that's what we're presenting here: Facts you can use to arm yourself when choosing the foods you choose and the goals you want to set.

We're not asking you to become like us—either of us! We're asking you to be yourself and absorb what we have learned.

It's not easy for many people to be themselves, because they're not sure who they are. That's the result of low self-esteem, in many ways. How to raise your self-esteem? Nothing succeeds like success. And the higher your self-esteem, the easier it is to just be yourself.

Diet is also a subtle form of torture. All right, it's not exactly like having your fingernails yanked out, or being tied to a chair and forced to listen to Barry Manilow records for a week. But it's not much fun, either. That's because most diets include another four-letter word that begins with "d": *deny*.

The principal thing you need to deny in your life is excessive fat. And the key to denying your body excess fat is to find a way you don't miss it at all.

Lower your weight, not your IQ.

Does dieting make you dumb? A study at the Institute of Food Research in Reading, England, tested seventy volunteers on everything from memory retention to mental processing. Those following major weight-loss diets fared so poorly that their performance sank to a level normally associated with normal people who had taken two stiff alcoholic drinks. The reason, according to the researchers, is that these dieters were suffering from a form of anxiety brought on by obsessing about food.

Why losing weight is a little like keeping your virtue.

Our grandmothers were familiar with a proverb that went: *Virtue is its own reward.* In other words, when things got hot and heavy with your boyfriend and you managed to keep saying "No" while your hormones were screaming *"Yes! Yes! Yes!,"* you were doing the right thing but didn't expect to get a medal for it.

Losing weight is a little like that. Do it for the reward and satisfaction it gives you, not because others insist on it.

Self-denial is indulgence of a propensity to forgo.
AMBROSE BIERCE

One of the weaknesses of traditional diets is that they ask you to abstain, which leads to minor mental anguish and a promise that you can reward yourself later with a "treat." Eat bland food, ignore hunger pains, change your eating habits cold turkey, and on the weekend you can maybe have a cookie. Yeah, right. Isn't that a little like the guy who kept banging his head against a wall because it felt so good when he stopped?

Here's our definition of the word, when it comes to losing weight:

DIET—a short-term form of self-torture, very popular among some cultures immediately after holidays and immediately before class reunions. Traditionally followed by a celebratory period of indulgence (see BINGE).

There's something else about starvation diets that few people realize.

Your body weight is made up primarily of fat and muscle (forget bones and the messy internal parts for a minute). People follow diets to lose fat from their bodies. So they reduce their calorie intake substantially, and prepare to suffer. But two things happen whenever you do this.

First, your body gets confused. "She's not giving me all the calories she used to," it decides. "Must be something serious going on, like famine. I'll slow down the metabolism and burn fewer calories than I normally do, until the famine's over and we're eating the foods we used to eat." Then it slips into a crisis mode to help you survive until you resume your normal eating habits. Unless you help your body resume its normal rate of metabolism with exercise or other physical effort, starving yourself doesn't have the initial impact on your weight that you expected. So you become frustrated. Which leads to a feeling of failure. Which leads to lower self-esteem. Which eventually leads to the to-hell-with-this-I'm-going-out-for-a-cheeseburger-and-fries syndrome.

Another thing happens that's really bizarre when you think about it.

If your body believes you're teetering toward starvation, its natural inclination is to survive. Any excess fat you've been storing is your body's long-term insurance for survival; you may need it somewhere down the road. But for now, you don't need all that muscle you've been carrying around. So that's what your body begins to feed on: muscle. Eventually it will get to your fat reserve. But by that time—unless you've been taking care to strike a balance in your plan to lose weight—your health is already suffering. And when you resume your normal eating habits, guess what your body does with the extra calories? *It makes new fat!* So here's the procedure:

1. You feel too fat, so you drastically reduce your calorie intake.

2. Your body thinks you're starving and begins burning up muscle.

3. You lose a little weight, grow frustrated with your diet, and resume your normal eating habits (98 percent do).

4. Your body turns the extra calories you are now eating into more fat.

5. You've starved yourself, lost some muscle mass, gone back to eating the things you used to eat, and now have more fat than you had when you started.

Is there a place for diet in your life? Of course there is. As long as the words "healthy" and "low-fat" are in front of it—not "starvation."

Besides, we have a revolutionary idea:

What if you were enjoying all the food you eat, eating as much of it as you want, and still seeing results? If that's the case, who needs a reward?

To paraphrase our dear old grannies: "Shopping for food while armed with knowledge about fat content is its own reward." It doesn't have quite the catchy rhythm of the original, but it works for us. You can continue to enjoy the texture and (most of) the flavor in foods you eat. The difference will be in the fat content of everything you put in your tummy. Remember that difference in measuring calories by weight: By the time your body processes a gram of protein or carbohydrates into a gram of fat, the calorie content is one-third less than it would have been had you eaten a gram of fat.

Is there a conspiracy to make you overweight?

Sometimes it seems that way. If you still believe there was a second assassin on the grassy knoll in Dallas or that Elvis is circling the earth in a flying saucer built by Howard Hughes, you can argue very convincingly that a bunch of food-company executives meet every month in a Rocky Mountain cabin and plan how to add inches to your waist and pounds to your hips.

Listen, it may be true.

But chances are it's not. Food-company executives aren't committed to making you fat. They're committed to making themselves

Eat now. We'll talk later.

Let's get this straight right away: We love food! And we assume you do as well. So stick with us and we promise you'll never feel the pangs of starvation while arming yourself against disease and health problems. In fact, here's what we each do to avoid hunger pangs:

Wendy: "I carry a feed bag."

It's true. When I'm jogging, traveling or working, I bring along foods that fill me up, provide some nourishment and are (almost) free of fat. I call it my "Feed Bag," and here are some of the things you're likely to find in it:

★ Pretzels

★ No Name Low-Fat Crispy Rice Marshmallow Squares

★ Baked potato chips

★ Air-popped popcorn

Barb: "Fruit and a batch of Chana."

I keep bananas and apples nearby, and I mix up a batch of Curried Chana now and then. It's a Trinidadian dish that's really delicious as a snack or as a side dish with chicken or in tortillas. Try it—here's the recipe:

1	can chick-peas	1
1	onion, chopped	1
2	cloves garlic, minced	2
1 tablespoon	(no more!) canola oil	15 mL
2 teaspoons	curry powder	10 mL
1 tablespoon	ketchup	15 mL
1 teaspoon	hot sauce	5 mL
	Salt and pepper	

Drain chick-peas; reserve ½ cup (125 mL) liquid. Sauté onion and garlic in oil. Add curry powder and cook 1 minute. Add chick-peas; cook 5 minutes. Add remaining ingredients, including reserved liquid. Simmer uncovered for 15 minutes, or until almost all liquid has evaporated. Store in a plastic bag.

rich by selling you what you want to eat. And if this means you want to eat more fat in your food than you need, whose fault is it?

Well, it's not entirely your fault. There's some blame to be spread around to places like the medical profession, the food packagers and the fitness industry.

We think doctors and nurses are terrific people. Really. They tend to be smart, hard-working and caring. Many of them literally work miracles every day. The biggest problem, when it comes to losing weight and staying fit, is that some members of the medical profession have underestimated our intelligence. If you ask basic questions such as "What's inside these pills that you're putting in my body?" or "Can I have a second opinion on that"?, the response is often: "Trust me, I'm a doctor."

We trust our mothers too, but when we play bridge with them we still cut the cards.

We envy and admire anyone who has the intelligence, ambition and energy to survive all the training it takes to become a physician. All that work and responsibility make the vast majority of doctors worth the fees they charge and the income they earn. But we should also remain aware of certain facts that have come to light in the past decade or so—not just about the medical profession, but about two more industries that thrive on the excess fat we consume.

Fact #1: Doctors aren't as smart about diets as they are about almost everything else, from hangnails to hernias. You may have heard this before, but it's still true and worth remembering:

On average, physicians, through all their years of training, receive about two and a half hours of classroom study on nutrition.[1] In other words, they spend more time discovering the location of the washrooms in the hospitals where they do their internship than they spend learning the intricacies of the foods we eat!

Fact #2: The fitness industry needs overweight people the way the FBI needs criminals. If everybody behaved like Mother Teresa, we'd have no cops, no judges, no courts, no

---

[1]John McDougall and Mary A. McDougall, *The McDougall Plan*, (Piscataway NJ: New Century, 1983), 7.

jails and no criminal lawyers. And if all of North America grew slim and fit tomorrow from eating low-fat and growing more active, millions of exercise machines would become boat anchors overnight and thousands of gyms would be silent and empty.

There's nothing wrong with working out in gyms, of course. Nothing wrong with those $3,000 fitness machines sold on TV at three o'clock in the morning either. Or with leaping around for six hours a week, trying to do jumping jacks in multipatterned leotards.

The point is, none of this is really necessary for overall fitness. You don't need the fitness clubs, the workout machines and the aerobic instructors. *But they need you.* Without you, they're out of business. Without your money, they're broke.

Fact #3: The food companies keep giving you what you want, not what you need. We're all logical people—well, most of the time. So when we go grocery shopping, we choose our food according to logical reasons. Is it a good price? Do we like the taste? Is it nutritional for us? Maybe, as we get older: Can I digest it easily? And if we still think they matter most: How many calories does it contain?

Excuse us, but did anybody ask about fat content?

More of us are beginning to, which is why food companies are putting the information on their labels. (They're also bowing to government regulations while doing it.) If we say we want it loud enough, we'll get it.

When you win, nothing hurts.
JOE NAMATH

Barb's Turn:

One thing that Wendy and I realized when we began planning this book is that a lot of weight problems are based as much on what people put *on* their foods as what they put *in* them. We're thinking of butter, margarine, mayonnaise and sour cream. They're all very high in fat content. There is more than enough fat inside most of the foods we eat—we shouldn't have to add more fat on top of them!

Bread without butter or marg may not be interesting. But you'll never miss it in a sandwich if the rest is made appealing and flavorful with things like thinly sliced onion, a dash of hot sauce or salsa, a dollop of mustard or horseradish, or something else to keep your taste buds from thinking about butter. Here's another idea: Fresh, homemade bread with no preservatives tastes wonderful as is. (If you can afford one, an automatic bread-making machine will change your bread-buying habits forever by ensuring you're eating low-fat bread, and you'll miss the butter even less.)

Instead of drizzling butter over hot vegetables such as Brussels sprouts, spinach and carrots, sprinkle them with lemon juice and sesame seeds. Can't eat baked potatoes without sour cream? No-fat sour cream is available in most supermarkets now. Add a sprinkle of lemon juice, some dried chives, and enjoy.

Salads—everybody thinks salads are healthy for them. Of course they are, but most salad dressings aren't, and that includes so-called Lite and Diet brands. You know what tastes as good as any fat-filled salad dressing and better than all the so-called calorie reduced brands? A microwaved mixture of two parts apple jelly and one part cider vinegar. (No microwave? Heat in a double-boiler.) Add a dash of celery salt and it's fabulous! And there's not a hint of fat in it.

So you don't need complicated recipes or substitutes to eliminate fat. Sometimes the best ideas are really very simple.

Hey, all you "superficial" cynics out there!

Whether you believe God created every creature on earth or that we all evolved from sea slugs, you have to ask yourself: What good is excess fat on your body?

Look around you—not at your friends and neighbors, but at other animals in the world. Who has fat? Whales, walruses and sea lions, that's who. But only because they need it! When you spend most of your life in water so cold that it breeds more icebergs than fish, you better wear a blubber overcoat. This goes, to a lesser extent, for ducks, geese and other animals who live without central heating and duvets. Fat serves a purpose for them. It helps them survive. It's as important as food, fur and feathers.

We mention this because some people still believe that fat is normal, that everyone concerned about slimming down is superficial, and that books like this one are just another sign of prejudice against overweight people.

Yes, there is prejudice against overweight people.

No, this book isn't about that. It's not about fads and fashions either. It's about your life, and how long you want to keep living it—and how well.

We'll assume you want to live a good life as long as possible. Who doesn't? It's generally agreed that the length of our lives is determined by three different factors:

1. Genetics. Or heredity, if you prefer. Choose parents who live long lives and you've boosted your chance of dancing jigs when you're in your nineties.

2. Fate. Nobody knows when a piano is going to slip out of a tenth-story window just as you're passing under it.

3. Lifestyle. This includes the foods you eat, the bad habits you avoid, and the tuning you give your body every now and then with healthful activity.

As you can see, two out of three things that can shorten or extend your life are in the hands of other people. Don't you think it makes sense to take charge of the third one—the only thing you can influence?

Many of you may be nodding at the wisdom of extending your years by taking charge of your own lifestyle. But maybe you're also thinking: "So what? I'll just settle for thinner thighs." Or: "I just want to be able to get back into my slacks again." Or: "This summer I want to walk on the beach without having the wrong parts jiggle at the wrong time."

Well, what's wrong with that?!

If those are some of the real reasons you're reading this book, don't you dare feel guilty about it. Most of all, don't let other people make you feel guilty about it. If somebody tells you that losing weight, eating low-fat and keeping fit is a fad or "so superficial," tell that person you're assuming command of the only aspect of life that affects your lifespan. Or, if you like, quote from this next part:

Eat this, morning, noon & night!

We have lots of low-fat recipes to come, but this is the kind of healthy snack that soothes hunger pangs. It makes about 6 servings, and each serving delivers 100 calories of energy, 28 grams of carbohydrates, 5 grams of protein and only 1 gram of fat!

Wendy and Barb's Quick Couscous Pudding

½ cup	couscous	125 mL
1 cup	skim milk	250 mL
¼ cup	raisins	60 mL
8 ounces	Astro French Vanilla Yogurt	250 mL
2 tablespoons	sugar (optional)	30 mL
	Ground cinnamon	

Heat milk just to the boiling point. Pour into a bowl with couscous, sugar (if using) and raisins. Stir well and set aside for 20 minutes. Blend with yogurt and sprinkle lightly with cinnamon. Serve warm or cold.

There's only one "ness" you need to focus on.

We all like labels. Labels make it easier to judge things and people, and they provide an excuse for not digging too far beneath the surface. This can be good or bad, as we'll see later, when we go shopping in the supermarket.

It's when we let the labels do all our thinking for us that we get into trouble.

For example, books like this one tend to get shelved under "Fitness" in stores and libraries. But we're not selling fitness here. There's nothing wrong with the word, except that it's a label that may turn people off. "Fitness" suggests sweaty bodies, Lycra shorts, expensive athletic shoes and a four-figure annual fee to join a club where they torture you with chrome-and-leather machines.

A lot of people like that stuff. A lot of people benefit from it. But that's not what we're talking about here.

You might think we're promoting "slimness" too, but that's not it either. Being slim is fine. Being too slim isn't. Slim doesn't necessarily translate into health or happiness. Forget slimness.

We're certainly not promoting madness—the diet madness that changes normally intelligent people into yo-yos who watch their weight drop while they torture themselves with starvation, watch it rise back to the same level it was before (or even higher) when they resume their old eating habits, then watch it plummet again and start a new round of guilt, starvation and madness.

The only "ness" we're interested in is "wellness." It's kind of an ungainly word, but it's the best one we know to describe what we're talking about. Wellness covers all the things that help you live a longer, happier life. Most of all, it lets you choose the activities that suit you, your body and your personal interests best.

Both of us believe in weight lifting. Correctly done, it tones your body, burns up fat and makes you feel a little . . . *dangerous.* If you're a woman, that's a nice feeling to have. Not because it means you can use a karate chop to crush the next goon who bothers you at a party, but because it adds to your overall self-confidence and self-esteem.

Percentage of all diseases in North America that are diet-related: 68 percent[2]

Here's Wendy Again:

We'll get into this in detail later, but I want to have a quick word with any women who are wincing at the idea of lifting weights. It won't turn your body into one big rippling muscle—not unless you want it to and have the basic body type needed. It won't give you arms that look like legs, either.

Weight lifting adds strength and firmness to your body in a way no other exercise can. Do it right and you won't even have to work up a sweat or invest in one of those torture machines.

I can bench-press my own weight, which was a goal I set for myself. Bench-pressing involves lying on your back and pushing upwards. It's great exercise for all the parts of your body above the waist.

So, whatever you do, please don't dismiss the idea of lifting weights as part of your wellness campaign. If it's not for you, fine. You can apply other techniques. But at least give it a try.

The other thing in your life that's tasty, exciting, colorful and important.

Sex.

Okay, so we used it to get your attention. But for the vast majority of humanity, sex is still up there with basic human needs—less important than eating, breathing and sleeping, and more important than trimming your toenails and watching *Seinfeld*.

---

[2]1988 U.S. Surgeon-General's Report on Nutrition & Health, #88-50210

So, assuming you still value, need, enjoy, and maybe even demand sex in your life, it's one more motive to care about the fat content in your meals and the physical shape of your body.

The first reason is self-evident: Sex and obesity do not go well together unless you and your partner are members of some bizarre fat-worshiping cult. If you're a woman with a weight problem, you almost certainly don't feel as sexually attractive as you did when you were slim . . . or as you will when you become slimmer. *Feeling attractive is a pretty basic part of feeling sexy.* If you think of yourself as a lump, or just lumpy, you're not going to fantasize yourself as a great lover. And you won't have any fantasies of reducing men—or at least your husband/ lover/partner—to shallow, drooling, pitiful fools at the mere sight of you. ("Is fantasy a major part of good sex?" you may ask. To which we reply: "Is fat a major part of lard?")

Perception is everything. If you perceive yourself as reasonably sexy and attractive, your libido will prance and wag its tail like a dog that wants you to toss it a bone. (Boy, did we get enough Freudian images in that sentence or what?)

Let's take a minute to face the truth about just one of the three billion or so differences between men and women. This one concerns staring back at themselves in a mirror when naked. Put a woman in front of a mirror with no clothes on and her response—at almost any stage in her life—usually goes something like this:

> *"Oh my God! Look at me! This is terrible!*
> *When did this happen? Why did this happen?*
> *I need to get on a diet! I need to get cosmetic surgery!*
> *I need to get dressed!"*

Put a naked man in front of the same mirror and he'll likely say:

> *"Hey, that's not bad. Pull in the tummy a bit,*
> *work out a little to tighten the pecs, maybe*
> *cut back on the beers this weekend, that's all*
> *I need. Besides, there's never too much of a good thing, right?"*

Marriage may have many pains, but celibacy has few pleasures.

DR. SAMUEL JOHNSON

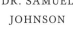

Risk of death from heart attack for the average North American male who eats meat regularly: 50 percent[3]
Risk of death from heart attack for the average North American male who consumes no meat: 15 percent[4]

Once you begin to both lose weight and firm up your body, you can expect a two-for-one payoff. First, you'll feel more attractive to others and more satisfied with yourself. Second, your partner—unless he has the sensitivity of a tree stump—will also notice the positive difference. Say what you will about intimacy, romance and all the other window dressing, physical appearance, which includes a firm body that's shaped in the right places, is still the champion pusher of men's "hot" buttons.

This second benefit of growing slim and firm—turning more men's eyes, and turning them farther than before—is a nice one to enjoy, as long as you're comfortable with your femininity. *But it's not the prime reason to change.* Do it for yourself. To change the way you feel about yourself. To improve your overall health and resistance to disease. To enjoy the sense of accomplishment you get from taking charge of your own life, in this small but important area at least.

Something else happens when you lose weight and become more physically fit: You enjoy both more sex and better sex. That's not just a promise or a come-on. It's a physiological, psychological, sociological fact. You want more sex and better sex? Get yourself healthy by pursuing wellness. And if you think the foods you eat have no effect on your body's performance both in and out of bed, you're wrong.

We were a little hard on doctors earlier, so it's time to make amends. We're especially grateful for doctors who recognize the importance of nutrition in the overall health of their patients, and

THE PERFECT HUSBAND
He tells you when you've got on too much lipstick/And helps you with your girdle when your hips stick.

OGDEN NASH

[3]W. Kannel, "Incidence and Prognosis of Unrecognized Myocardial Infarction—An Update on the Framingham Study," *New England Journal of Medicine,* 311 (1984), 1144.
[4]R. Philips, "Coronary Heart Disease—Differing Dietary Habits: A Preliminary Report," *American Journal of Clinical Nutrition* 31 (1978), 181.

one of them has written a very good book titled *Sexual Nutrition*. Here's what the good doctor, who specializes in both sexuality and diet, has to say about the subject:

> Sexual dysfunction is a degeneration of body parts. It can encompass a number of different organs or systems, including the mind, nerves, genitals, endocrine glands or blood vessels. Diet-related problems that commence in the twenties or thirties and steadily increase into the forties and fifties and later ages are often tied to over-eating, improper selection of foods and lack of exercise.[5]

He's referring to all the complex actions and reactions our bodies experience during sex, and this is neither the time nor the place to examine them. But if nothing else, a lighter and tighter body is going to have more energy to perform whatever physical exertion you need to enhance your sex life. If "breathing hard" once meant sexual excitement to you, and it now describes what happens when you walk from the sofa for another bowl of potato chips, you should be getting the message here. Or to put it another way: Imagine tying a fifty-pound sack of flour around your waist and trying to have sex at the same time. Now imagine cutting the rope and watching that sack fall away to the floor.

Increased risk of breast cancer for women who eat meat daily compared with women who eat meat less than once a week: 3.8 times higher[6]

Increased risk of fatal prostate cancer for men who consume meats, dairy products and eggs daily compared with men who eat them sparingly: 3.6 times higher[7]

---

[5]Morton Walker, *Sexual Nutrition* (Garden City, NY: Avery, 1994), 128.
[6]Takeshi Hirayama, paper presented at the Conference on Breast Cancer and Diet, U.S.–Japan Cooperative Cancer Research Program, Fred Hutchinson Center, Seattle, WA, March 14–15, 1977.
[7]P. Hill, "Environmental Factors of Breast and Prostatic Cancer," *Cancer Research* 41 (1981), 3817.

We've had fun with sex, life and the whole darn thing here, but it's a serious matter. A better sex life won't necessarily make you a happier, healthier, more fulfilled person. But happy, healthy, fulfilled people invariably have a satisfactory sex life.

The connection should be obvious.

Now let's tell stories, then start getting *Armed and Dangerous.*

We've taken this long to set the stage for becoming *Armed and Dangerous* because we want you to recognize two things:

Losing excess fat is important to your entire well-being, including not just how long you live, but how well you live.

Losing excess fat can be fun. It *should* be fun, and it will be fun.

Even when they're told that eating low-fat and keeping fit are both important and fun, some people remain skeptical about their own ability to achieve success. We understand. But we ask you to read about our situations as they were not so long ago, and compare them with your own. Then we'll help you have as much fun, and produce the same dramatic results, as we did.

Check off these facts if you agree with them:

❏ Most diets are failures, and the blame belongs, not with the dieter, but with diets themselves.

❏ I don't want to be someone else's idea of me; I just want to be a healthier, happier me.

❏ If I starve myself, I'll lose muscle before I lose fat; when I resume my eating habits, I'll have less muscle and more fat than when I began. This is known as a loser's game.

❏ I don't need expensive machines to lose weight and tone up.

❏ It's nobody's business but mine if I want to lose weight for strictly aesthetic reasons.

❏ Sex is better with less fat around.

If you don't agree with a statement above, write your reasons here:

_____

_____

_____

_____

_____

_____

CHAPTER THREE

Wendy's Story: Did I Really Deserve This?

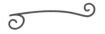

All young children love Christmas. When I was a very young girl, I think I loved Christmas even more than others because I felt that, in one small way, I was more closely connected to the joy it brought thousands of people.

About a month before Christmas Day, my parents would drive me and my sister to Toronto to view the famous Santa Claus Parade. We would rise early in the morning and my mother would bundle us against the cold because we would be standing at the curb for hours, waiting for the parade to begin, and then watching it pass, screaming in laughter and joy.

The parade always seemed to be miles long, crowded with floats, clowns, horses, marching bands, majorettes and, finally, the arrival of Santa Claus himself. He always received the biggest cheer, of course. And while I was as happy as anyone else to see him and hear him laugh and wish everyone a "Merry Christmas," I knew Santa's arrival marked something else as well.

It meant the Christmas window in Eaton's department store would finally be unveiled.

Every year, Eaton's giant store in downtown Toronto devoted its largest display windows to a Christmas animated scene. No one knew in advance what the theme would be; it was always a closely guarded secret. For days, the display windows were shrouded in heavy curtains while the panorama was prepared. When Santa took his throne in Eaton's toy department, it signaled the official unveiling of that year's window. Every day from then until Christmas, the crowds at the Eaton's Christmas window were so deep they spanned the entire width of the sidewalk, forcing pedestrians to walk in the street.

The Christmas display windows grew more elaborate each year, with their animation and complex staging. One year there might be a forest scene with bears turning their heads majestically, rabbits hopping in and out of holes, mice skittering here and there across the snow, and perhaps an owl peeking from behind a branch high up in the trees. The next year it could be a re-creation of Santa's North Pole workshop, with quarreling elves and more pesky mice and Rudolph peeking through the window.

The competition to make Eaton's Christmas window more elaborate and enticing every year was driven by the fact that the store's biggest competitor, Simpson's department store, had a similar animated display directly across the street. The two retailing giants vied with each other to lure the biggest audience—and, of course, the most shoppers.

But only Eaton's display window attracted me. Not because it was the original, or even because it was the most ornate—most years, it was a toss-up between the two stores—but because the animated animals, toys and settings were all created by my father, who worked for the company that produced the animated scenes for Eaton's. All the people laughing and pointing and enjoying themselves were being entertained by my father's handiwork.

I would stand there, barely able to peer over the window ledge into this fantastic wonderland where it was always joyful and exciting, and know it was the product of my father's skills and imagination. Naturally, I believed at least a little bit of it was made especially for me. All the other small kids who were "Oooohing" and "Aaaahing" or just standing with their mouths open could enjoy it too. But I felt a special ownership.

I felt gifted and rewarded.

After my parents finally pulled me away from the window, we would drive to my uncle Ray's house in Toronto for a great family feast. Ray was my mother's brother, and their relationship defined the closeness of everyone else in my family when I was a small child. My parents were Scottish immigrants, and among the qualities they brought with them to Canada was an appreciation for hard work. Nothing significant came easily, in their view. Hard work wasn't just necessary; it was a validation of your worth as a person.

If you think they were always serious and dour, forget that stereotype of Scots. I recall those family feasts being filled with laughter and jokes, and though the food was fairly simple and out of fashion now—Sundays meant roast beef and Yorkshire pudding with hot gravy and potatoes—there was always plenty of it.

But I remember, too, that when all the family was wrapped up in their celebration of being together, my mind's eye would return

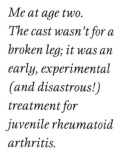

Me at age two. The cast wasn't for a broken leg; it was an early, experimental (and disastrous!) treatment for juvenile rheumatoid arthritis.

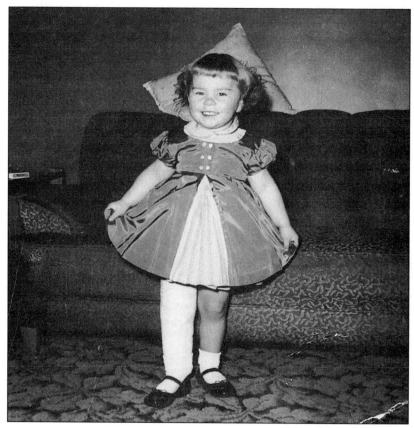

to the department store downtown, and once again I would be peering through the window at my father's imaginary world, where it never rained and no one ever cried because they suffered from near-constant, excruciating pain or because other children teased them for having one leg shriveled and shorter than the other.

Like me.

I was the oldest of three girls, and I suppose I filled all the expectations of "The Oldest Child": serious, determined and protective of my younger sisters. One sister, Jan, is three years younger than I, but there's a gulf of thirteen years between me and Lori, the youngest.

My mother was and still is a beautiful woman. Long before working mothers became almost fashionable and necessary, she held a full-time job. The work ethic was drilled into us at a very early age. As soon as I was deemed old enough, I was expected to start preparing dinner immediately after school and to have it ready for my parents' arrival home. Saturday mornings were cleaning time. My mother, Jan and I tackled the dusting, washing, waxing and generally tidying-up without question. It simply had to be done, and that was that.

My family also operated a small lodge in cottage country during the summer months. When school was finally out in June, I traveled to the lodge with my grandmother and stayed until Labor Day. Naturally, there was work to be done and I was expected to pitch in and do my share, whether it was baby-sitting or helping to paint the cabins. But there was also fun to be had, and I found all the time I needed to go boating, fishing, water-skiing and hiking.

This sounds so out-of-date, doesn't it? It may seem difficult for younger people to grasp that we were a nuclear, normal, *functional* family. We worked hard and took as much enjoyment from our labor as we could. We respected one another, especially those who were older than us. We felt safe from danger, which always seemed far away. And we assumed this was the way things should always be, *would* always be.

It sounds idyllic, and for a time it was. The problem I faced—

the only problem, I suppose—was one of constant pain, which diluted and corroded all the joy I should have felt as a young girl in this warm environment.

My mother first realized I had a problem when I was about eighteen months old. I would wake up crying, literally screaming in pain. When my mother took me for a walk, I had trouble maintaining even the slowest pace. One day, after noticing that one of my knees was swollen each morning, she took me to our family doctor, who prescribed special treatment: five ASA tablets a day and several months with my affected leg in a cast, which immobilized it completely.

I don't remember the immediate results, of course. But my mother recalls vividly the sight of my leg when the cast was finally removed. The muscles had atrophied almost completely. Things were worse than ever, and I was sent to spend eight months in a children's hospital for treatment. By the time I was released, just before my third birthday, my life had changed in two ways: I had a new baby sister and one leg substantially shorter than the other.

My parents finally had an accurate diagnosis of my condition: juvenile rheumatoid arthritis.

We tend to think of arthritis as a disease suffered primarily by elderly people, but of course it can strike much earlier—in my case, as early as a year and a half. The effects of arthritis can range from the merely annoying to the totally crippling, and it's associated with a wide range of causes, from infection and trauma to gout and bursitis.

As a young girl, I didn't care what the disease was or why I was suffering from it. I just knew the pain it caused was always there and, according to the medical specialists of the day, it would be there for the rest of my life. By the time I began school, my afflicted leg was a full inch and a half shorter than the other. On a five-year-old this is a major difference, and I walked as though I had one leg on the sidewalk and the other in the gutter.

To help correct it, my mother bought me special shoes with one built-up sole. Along with my lurching walk and inability to run, the shoes made me the object of jokes from the other children. Mom remembers me returning home from school day after day, always in tears, embarrassed by the teasing I suffered from other children. I hated the disease I had, hated the funny shoes I had to wear, and hated the pain I was suffering and the medications I had to take to control it.

My parents did all they could to make me feel protected and loved, and I thank them for that. But the rest of the world wasn't as gentle with me. When you are five years old, in almost constant pain and unable to do what other five-year-olds can do, it has a deep effect on you. In my case, it made me somewhat shy and self-conscious—which will come as a major surprise to anyone who has seen Barb and me conduct our seminars or appear on network television shows!

Fortunately (according to my mother), I managed to retain a fairly happy disposition. Good thing—I would certainly need it.

When I was six, some well-meaning doctors suggested a solution for my shorter leg. They would open up my knee and put plastic spacers in between the bones. At least that's the way my mother recalls it. To her credit, she refused the idea. I don't know how well it might have worked (I shiver a little just thinking about the idea now—an inch and a half of plastic separating the joints of my knee?!), but I began to learn one of the important lessons of my life from that point.

You see, when my parents chose not to have the operation performed, they decided to simply ignore my shorter leg and encourage me to lead as normal a life as possible. Why let a leg that's an inch and a half shorter than the other prevent me from doing what other kids my age were doing? Naturally, they over-compensated—which was, in hindsight, a brilliant thing to do.

So, there I was, the little girl with the gimpy leg and a perma-nent case of rheumatoid arthritis taking *dancing lessons*! And *baton twirling*! And *accordion lessons*. Okay, the accordion lessons didn't do a lot for my legs (although hanging that thing on my chest every day probably strengthened my back). But all the dancing and high-stepping had an effect on the disease and my leg. Staying active seemed to hold the pain at bay, and the exercise may have stimulated my short leg enough to encourage it to grow.

Whatever it was, over the next ten years the difference between the lengths of my legs eventually disappeared. Heavy doses of my medication helped control the pain that was always there, lurking in the background. So I entered my mid-teens with a reasonably balanced body and a fairly positive outlook—important qualities for a teenage girl. I was still basically a shy person, which I tried to overcome by being more of a tomboy than my girlfriends. I was the auburn-haired, freckle-faced class clown, the kid who always had a new joke to tell, and who loved making other people laugh.

Not surprisingly, I was not a very good student in high school. I had inherited something of a creative outlook from my father, but I thought I would enjoy working with people instead of mechanical things like he did. In my mid-teens, I was interested in three things above all: boys, music and hair styling. So I was determined, as soon as I was old enough and brave enough, to become a hairdresser and probably get married.

That's about when the next major pain encounter arrived. (See now why I reject that "No pain, no gain" nonsense?)

I was fourteen years old and paying a routine visit to my dentist one day when he looked me in the eye with a solemn expression on his face. I thought he was going to lecture me about not brushing correctly, but instead he told me that my lower jaw had stopped growing. Just like that. My bite was shrinking and my jaw had receded noticeably. The condition, known as Still's disease, is related to arthritis. I'm sure this isn't the medical description, but I've always had the feeling that when we beat the arthritis in my legs the disease said, "I'll fix you guys." Then it broke camp in my legs and headed for a more prominent location: my neck and lower jaw.

In fact, even before the dentist noticed my smaller bite and jaw difficulties, I had been growing aware of increasing stiffness in my neck. When I needed to look left or right, I found it easier to turn my entire upper body in that direction instead of just my head.

That was serious enough, but the doctors were more concerned about correcting my jaw and restoring my profile to the way it should be. So an operation was planned and the procedure explained to me in all its gory detail.

(Warning—if some aspects of surgery make you uncomfortable, you may want to skip the next few paragraphs. If you choose to read the details, imagine how it felt to be a basically shy fourteen-year-old, hearing for the first time what the doctors planned to do to you.)

The corrective surgery consisted of breaking my jaw (*Crack!*), pulling it forward (*Yank!*), wiring it in place through my teeth (*Sproing!*) and leaving it that way for three months (*Yikes!*). That sounded drastic enough, but they had more plans. Two 2-inch cuts would be made under each ear and along the jaw line. My lower jaw would be cut and plastic spacers inserted to extend it so the two jaws met correctly. (I had visions of a demonic surgeon from ten years earlier rubbing his hands together and saying, "So you wouldn't put the spacers in your knee, huh? Well, we'll put 'em in your mouth instead. How d'ya like *that*?") I also would need four teeth removed and have to wear braces for several months.

The doctors tried to make me feel better by saying I would be only the seventh person in Canada to have this type of surgery performed on them. Maybe they assumed being seventh would make me feel lucky. It didn't. I would rather have been the ten-thousandth.

I lived on nothing but liquids and baby food for those three months following the operation, while my family continued to enjoy roast beef and Yorkshire pudding each Sunday. I don't know what was more torturous—the pain of the operation, or the aroma of food I loved but was incapable of eating.

I looked forward to the day when the wires through my gums would be removed. Unfortunately, I was given no anesthetic before the procedure, and I still remember the excruciating pain as the wires were pulled through my gums. The incisions along my jaw line healed well, but there was more to be done.

The following year, a small crescent-shaped piece of silicon was inserted in my chin through an incision inside my mouth, below the lower lip. (This is the first time I have publicly admitted that I have a silicon implant. Of course, there's only one, and it's a little higher than the usual location for women my age.)

All in all, the surgery was successful, but complications remain almost thirty years later. The operation created a deep-seated fear of dentists that I can't overcome, and my jaw opening is still restricted. As a result, I have endured more than my share of cavities, extractions and root-canal work—even with the help of my patient, gifted and understanding dentist.

At sixteen, feeling a little better about my appearance and dating my high-school sweetheart, I quit school and began working for the same company as my mother during the day, attending hairdressing school at night.

My mother suffered along with me through all those years. She was diagnosed with arthritis around the time of my birth. Her lovely hands grew swollen and riddled with pain, and I have vivid memories of driving her to the doctor for injections of cortisone and anti-inflammatory drugs, shot directly into her knuckles without anesthetic of any kind. She would emerge from the doctor's office saying nothing and speaking as little as possible all the way home, before rushing into her bedroom and closing the door behind her. Once I followed her and, opening the door, discovered her sobbing in agony by herself—she refused to let her children know the pain she was suffering.

In spite of that memory, my image of my mother through all those years consists of an attractive woman whose hair was always perfectly coiffed and whose makeup was impeccably applied. To this day, I don't fully understand how she did it. But her independence, her strength and her unashamed concern for her appearance still leave me in awe.

I followed the principal lesson of my Scots heritage—"Hard work never hurt anybody"—by taking two jobs while attending hairdressing school several miles away in Toronto four nights a week and all day Saturday. Even today, I grow exhausted thinking about my routine: Working in a plant cafeteria from 8:00 A.M. to 4:00 P.M., driving to Toronto to attend hairdressing school until 10:00 P.M., then working with my fiancé cleaning offices from midnight to 3:00 A.M. Only a determined seventeen-year-old could maintain that kind of schedule, and I was both seventeen and determined.

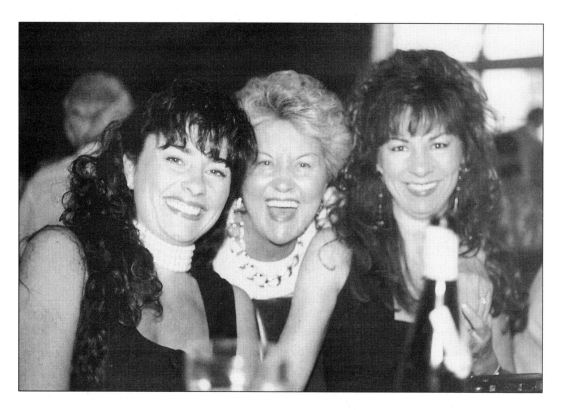

The result of all this hard work was mixed. I graduated from hairdressing school with honors, married my high-school sweetheart, acquired a new sports car and motorcycle for us, and purchased a brand-new town house, where we installed a mini-salon in the back. My husband and I took exotic vacations, and I began building a loyal clientele for my business. Determined to expand my horizons, I continued my education with Spanish lessons, art studies and courses in business management and accounting.

The fantasy house-with-the-white-picket-fence had come true and, several years later, as I entered my mid-twenties, the only thing missing was a baby.

Nice idea. Bad timing.

First, all those years of maintaining two jobs and attending hairdressing school were hardly the best treatment for my arthritis. I managed to control the pain with medication, but the older I grew, the more difficult the chore became.

Here I am with my sister Lori (left) and my mom (center). Check out their low-fat recipes!

Second, my marriage, born in the confidence and energy of youth, was beginning to crumble around me.

In spite of those problems—or maybe because of them—I remember the first few months of my pregnancy as a time when I felt better than I had in years. Then, in my fifth month, two dramatic events occurred.

First my grandmother passed away after a long and valiant fight against cancer. The memories of my days with her at the summer camp became even more precious to me. A few days after her funeral, a drunk driver crossed over to my lane and we collided head-on at high speed. I emerged with lacerations on my legs and forehead, a totally destroyed sports car, and some paranoia about driving that's still almost as deep as my fear of dentists.

After that, giving birth was almost easy. Hey, it was *very* easy—within four hours of the first contraction, and without an epidural, I was holding a beautiful seven-pound, six-ounce boy in my arms. Lee became, and still is, the apple of my eye and a major source of much joy . . . okay, and some consternation, now that he's a teenager!

A week after Lee's arrival, I began experiencing pain in my right side. It grew to excruciating levels, and I was rushed to hospital suffering, the doctors first assumed, an attack of appendicitis. The eventual diagnosis proved more complicated. My right kidney had become severely infected due to being crushed during my pregnancy, the result of being located in an abnormally low position in my body. What's more, my urethra had grown clogged with kidney stones. The kidney had to come out.

No major problem, I was told. Our bodies can survive very well, thank you, with one functioning kidney. My doctor assured me the operation would be routine—a few hours under general anesthetic, a week or so to recoup my strength, a small scar on my back, and things would be back to normal. The trouble is, my definition of "normal" was different from others'.

Complications began when the anesthetist was unable to feed the tube down my throat, thanks to my restrictive jaw opening. This required an emergency tracheotomy, which meant cutting into my windpipe below the larynx. Once the operation was under way, the surgeons discovered my urethra was so badly damaged that they had to replace a section of it with plastic tubing. So I woke up to discover I was breathing through an opening at the base of my neck with a two and a half foot incision across my body closed with thin wire zigzagged through both sides. There was more. A drainage opening from the urethra operation leaked into a plastic bag, and every two hours a nurse arrived to clear my breathing tube with a suction device and keep me from suffocating.

Three weeks later I returned home literally a different woman, and began living a different kind of life.

D octors warn patients to expect complications when recovering from major surgery like the one I had just gone through. In my case, the complications were a little unusual: Instead of spending the next few months restoring my energy, I had to invest the time in dissolving my marriage. My husband and I worked on the separation agreement and negotiated the sale of our possessions and my white-picket-fence dream home. After nine months (a bitter coincidence after becoming a mother, don't you think?), we emerged as two separated people prepared to carry on separate lives. Of course, mine was a little complicated by the fact that I was now a single mother with a fast-growing baby boy and no child support.

I'm trying hard to put the best light on things here, but the fact is I entered a very difficult period in my life. On the bright side, I was fairly active, still in my mid-twenties; my baby was healthy; and I had a vocation. Not so bad.

On the other side, I was a single working mother at a time when that phrase was still unfashionable. My earnings were lower than they were when my ex-husband and I had been partners, and my expenses were substantially higher. By the time I'd paid various debts and struggled through the first year trying to raise Lee on my own, all the assets of my marriage were gone. Soon I was living in a run-down tenement in a terribly rough part of town with no car and no savings. The hours when I wasn't working at the salon were spent protecting Lee from various social threats, maintaining my sanity (especially through the "Terrible Twos" period of his life) and keeping my spirits up.

On Saturday nights we counted the cockroaches climbing the wall behind my used TV set and tried to ignore the noise of domestic battles raging in neighboring apartments. Sunday mornings I would place Lee in his little wagon for a trip to the park—a trip that began by pulling him down a darkened hallway and hearing the glass from shattered light bulbs crunch beneath my feet and the wagon wheels. Then we'd ride down in the elevator to the ground floor together, holding our noses against the stench of urine.

Single mothers in the poorer parts of town go through this every day of their lives. I suppose, in my case, I felt the loss more acutely because I thought I had done all the "right" things. I had worked hard, tried to be strong and independent, and maintained a positive outlook. I had tasted all the fruits of that hard work with a sports car, vacations, a fine wardrobe and a beautiful home. The loss of these material things was bad enough, but I had also lost both companionship and the social status of being that rare and exotic creature: a young, successful wife and career woman.

Actually, I'd lost even more than that. My family was spread out by now. Even my parents had divorced, and my mother and youngest sister were living far away, in warm, sunny Florida. My sister Jan had married and moved away to Alberta, where she had started her own family, with two girls and a boy. I missed them all so much, but there was no way I could afford to travel and visit them on my own.

In fact, if it hadn't been for Lee, the pain from my arthritis and the cockroaches behind the TV set, I'd have had no companions at all.

I hit bottom, I suppose, the day my ex-husband arrived to take Lee with him for Christmas dinner. So there I was, the little girl whose daddy had created all the magic in Eaton's window and made thousands of people happy, sitting home alone at Christmas in a run-down high-rise. I thought I might as well make use of my time. So I opened a can of floor wax and a bottle of Drambuie. For the next hour I'd wax the floor, have a drink, cry a bit, apply a little more wax, take another drink, and start the whole cycle over again. Merry Christmas, I told myself. Pour the wax, rub it in,

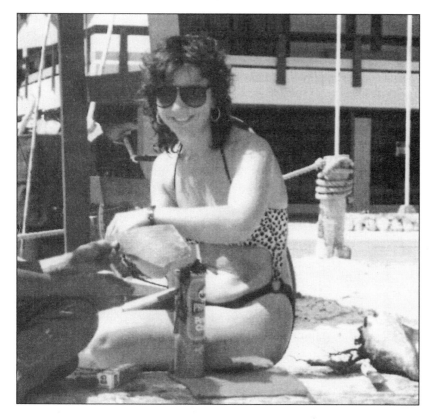

Me as a single mother—before I discovered low-fat eating and fitness training. When I was a teenager, this isn't quite what "letting it all hang out" meant.

take a drink, dry the tears, buff the floor. Pour the wax, rub it in, take a drink. (For God's sake don't get them mixed up—you know what Drambuie does to a floor?!)

Things, I told myself, could not possibly get worse.

Naturally, they did.

Two floors above me, another woman was feeling even more pain. Much more pain. Or maybe she wasn't fortunate enough to be able to draw on some inner source of strength. I'll never know, but I do know that it became too much for her. She threw herself from her apartment, and I glanced up just in time to see her fall past my window.

The rest of the tragedy played out like a familiar television show. Police and ambulances arrived amid screaming sirens and flashing lights. Spectators gathered with horrified expressions. Witnesses were interviewed by police and news reporters. Finally, the blood was washed away, the vehicles departed to wait for the next victim, the neighbors returned to their homes, and life went on.

I watched it all from my window. It's a lesson, I told myself, and the lesson is: Never let yourself get so far down that it comes to this. Change your life.

I'd like to say that my neighbor's suicide was enough stimulation to start changing my life immediately. Instead, it began a slow process that is only now paying off, fifteen years later.

Eventually I agreed to form a partnership with a male hairdresser, and we launched a business called "Shear Artistry." I was earning less than $200 a week and still receiving no support money from Lee's father, but it was a beginning. Lee and I moved to a small town house with a private yard, I bought an old jalopy for me and a bicycle for Lee, and the long climb began.

One of the biggest hurdles to overcome was raising my self-esteem. I don't believe in self-pity and, believe me, none is intended in telling this tale. I may have experienced sadness, loneliness, anger, depression and all those other emotions that single mothers who live on the edge of poverty (or deep within it) know all too well. But self-pity achieves nothing.

Self-esteem, of course, is something else. Everyone needs it, the more the better. Mine was at a very low point. Things were better in some ways—my son and I were living in a safer, more secure environment—but worse in others.

I hadn't totally shed the weight gained from my pregnancy, and between the long hours spent at work (cutting hair six days a week, doing bookkeeping chores on Sunday) and spending time with my son, I had precious little time to devote to myself. I felt unattractive, uninteresting and unappealing. I was lonely, and in almost constant pain from my worsening arthritic condition. The only person who seemed interested in my life was my married business partner, so I tended to pour out my melancholy thoughts to him. He was caring and attractive, and we were together ten or twelve hours a day.

You can guess what happened next.

The romance was as bittersweet as you might expect. I spent most of my working hours with my lover during the day, then went home alone to be with my son at night and on weekends.

My youngest sister's arrival from Florida was a major turning point in my life. She was determined to follow the same career I had, and soon I was playing the role of both sister and mother (remember, she's thirteen years younger than I am). Soon she was qualified, and Lori joined my partner and I at our newest salon location, where we added a new twist to the hairdressing business—a separate salon for children only, which we called "Kiddy Kutters." Youngsters could play games and watch videos while waiting to have their hair cut as they sat astride wooden horses instead of in normal chairs.

For five years, I settled into a routine of caring for my son, working long hours at the salon and trying to avoid feeling lonely and deprived. Lori, Lee and I made our own inexpensive fun. We danced to old records on Friday nights, walked in the park on Sunday afternoons, and watched every penny's worth of expenses when we went shopping for food or clothing.

It was the frugal shopping that got us into the most trouble.

During all those years, we never went to a movie or ate at a good restaurant. More and more, our lives revolved around the foods we cooked and ate in my town house. Food was comfort. Food was escape. Food was fun.

But too much of the food was fat.

We devoured peanut butter, cookies, nuts, pastries, cake mixes, cheese, pork chops, butter, potato chips, puddings, whipped cream—the works. Eventually Lori and I were delighted to discover that we could share each other's clothes. Hey, that was fun! Thirteen years apart and we were both the same size!

The bad news, of course, was that we both weighed 160 pounds. I was 5 feet, 4 inches tall, Lori was 5 feet, 2 inches, and all the clothes we shared were size 16. Something had to give besides the seams.

It's not really an excuse, but I was facing many demands by then. Doctors had prescribed Ritalin to control my son's hyperactivity, and the price of my arthritis medicine simply skyrocketed. Both prescriptions ate up large chunks of my income. (As a self-employed person, I had no drug plan.) Just to put me a little closer to the edge, I grew prone to kidney infections. These can severely damage your kidneys, and of course I don't carry a spare. Several times the agonizing pain from my kidney would wake me in the middle of the night, and I would follow a familiar procedure: Wake Lori, ask her to care for Lee, call a cab and rush to the hospital for treatment. Afterwards I'd be faced with a round of expensive antibiotics and harshly instructed by doctors to "Take it easy."

Thank you, doctor. But running a business, caring for a hyperactive child, living from hand to mouth, and watching your life pass in a haze of sixteen-hour working days and the side effects of painkillers was as easy as I could take it.

In spite of the hard work, the two salon locations we operated in commercial malls and my careful scrutiny of expenses, I grew no farther ahead financially than when I began. Just to make things worse, the romance with my partner had run its course. It was time to change my life again.

I found a lovely old Victorian home near an upscale residential area and took the plunge. Managing to purchase it at an attractive price (I sold my car for the down payment) and finding a bank manager who trusted me to make the mortgage payments, I set to work redecorating the place myself, converting it into a special location where customers felt cozy and comfortable. Then I rented a nearby one-bedroom apartment (I had to walk to work), Lori found a place of her own, I called my new business "Hampshire House Hair," and I was on my way.

But to where? Here's the picture:

I was thirty-six years old, forty pounds overweight, financially strapped to the limit, raising a child on my own without support money, and spending more money on medications and physiotherapy to control my pain than on almost any other item on my shopping list. I was so lethargic that I could barely walk up a flight of stairs. I ate what and when I could. I grew depressed. I grew fat. I grew almost helpless.

If the arthritis, kidney infections and other health problems were wearing me down this much in my mid-thirties, how would I ever survive my forties? What would happen to me in my fifties? Would I ever make it to sixty?

Larger and larger doses of painkilling medication weren't the answer. There had to be something else.

And thank goodness there was.

What does a lonely, overweight, overworked woman do when she's not working, caring for her child or watching TV? Well, she can always look at other people's bodies, especially if they're better than hers.

So, I'm flipping through *Muscle & Fitness* one day, and there it is: The story of a woman my age who has suffered from arthritis all her life. Boy, did we have something in common! (She also suffered from anorexia, which we clearly did *not* have in common....) Her cure was simple and effective: She changed to a low-fat, high-protein diet; and she put that protein to work by building and strengthening the muscles around her aching joints. The new, stronger muscles provided better support, subduing the arthritic pain.

It couldn't be that simple, could it? But it was.

It all began to make sense to me. I'd been shopping for food without regard for its content. If it was cheap and I liked the taste, in the cart it went.

For years, I had been treating the *effect* of my arthritis—the pain in so many of my joints—instead of treating the *cause*. Arthritis weakens your joints; stronger muscles help compensate for the weakness.

I was so excited that I called Lori, who had remarried and moved to Florida. (Did I tell you Lori was first married at seventeen, just like Jan and me? Did I tell you that all three marriages failed? Do you see a pattern here?) "You won't believe all the low-fat foods we have down here!" Lori said when I told her I was changing my diet. "Come on down, spend a few days in the sun, and we'll get you started."

Look, this wasn't a miracle cure. I have to be honest here. What takes me a paragraph or two to describe actually occurred over a few months. *But I felt the difference almost from the beginning!*

Reducing my fat intake to less than 25 percent of total calories was enough to melt inches from my waist. Lifting weights and finding fun ways to exercise built muscle tone, which reduced the swelling and pain from over forty years of arthritis. Cutting back on pain medication made me feel more alert, more alive and more

Okay, this one I can look at without grimacing. And it didn't take nearly as much denial, self-discipline or hard work as you think. In fact, most of it was fun!

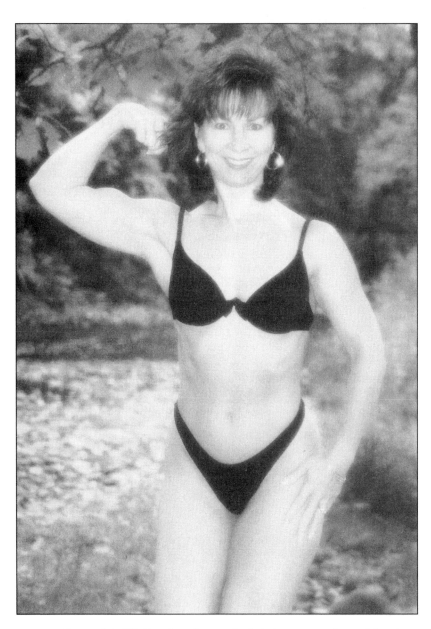

prepared to tackle life head-on instead of sitting around watching it beat me up.

The reduction in both my weight and level of pain made me feel almost euphoric. Talk about positive feedback! But I think I hit the pinnacle the day I easily bench-pressed my own weight.

Instead of the woman who just a few months earlier couldn't raise her own spirits, I had become a woman who was now raising metal barbells that weighed as much as she did!

By the way, I didn't develop rippling biceps and a washboard stomach from lifting weights. I don't look like one of those shiny and lumpy hulks you see on the covers of the weight-lifting magazines. I wasn't interested in that. I was only interested in feeling and looking normal. Frankly, I think I did better than normal.

Here's where you have to trust me, because what I'm about to say is totally true, and the primary reason for doing this book:

When I changed the foods I eat and the shape of my body, everything else in my life began to change. It was almost as though I was watching it happen to someone else. Psychologists are probably not surprised by this, nor are experienced fitness trainers, who see it all the time with their best clients. But until it happens to you, you can't imagine the difference that changing your body can make to your mind.

Do you really think that looking good, dressing well and fitting into a smaller wardrobe is merely "superficial"?

Do you really believe that a fortyish woman who enjoys turning men's heads when wearing a bikini at the beach is shallow?

Do you really think that doing whatever it takes to make you feel more comfortable about yourself is self-centered?

If you do, you're very mistaken. So stop thinking that way.

Whatever you do that is true to yourself and healthy for your self-esteem is worth the effort.

Think about the real benefits I earned from discovering my low-fat "cruise control" setting, and the rewards of exercise.

I reduced my level of painkillers dramatically. In fact, I go for long periods without needing any at all. *Do not for a moment believe that even the safest, most effective painkillers don't produce some long-term residual effects on your body.* They do. So whatever you can do to eliminate them improves your health.

I learned to handle stress better—all the stress that any working single mother feels. Why? Because I felt more relaxed, more content, more comfortable with myself, and *more confident in my strength to deal with stressful situations.* Stress has many causes, and one is the belief that you are not in control of your own life. (It's also a proven cause of most depression.)

Among all the good things that happened when I became Armed and Dangerous *was meeting my sweet, gentle partner, Bill.*

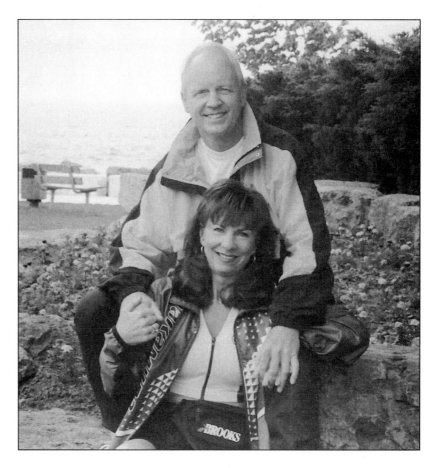

I had never considered myself a writer, but my success inspired me so much that I dashed off an article about my experience and sent it to *Muscle & Fitness*—who published it along with a picture of me in a bikini. Wow! Now I'm a published author and a pinup, all at once!

I discovered my success was contagious. My son, Lee, impressed with the positive effects of body-building and healthy eating on his mother, began to lift weights and change his eating habits. Hey, that was kind of neat, having a teenage son following in his mother's footsteps, so to speak. Soon something even neater happened: His own self-esteem soared, along with his marks at school.

And I can't prove a direct connection between the woman I became and the man I met soon after. But I believe it exists. Now I share my life with the kindest, most gentle man I have ever known, and our relationship restored faith in love and romance that I hadn't felt since my teenage years.

In a way, all my success with low-fat eating and simple keep-fit exercises went to my head. I became a kind of low-fat/keep-fit/born-again evangelist. I wanted everyone I met to share my discovery. I collected articles from magazines and books that promoted a healthy lifestyle. I'd take a break from styling my customers' hair to demonstrate body-building moves.

I would tell them the same thing I'm telling you here. You don't have to make a total change in your life. Start with a small change, watch the effect it has on you, and draw strength from it to make more changes, bit by bit. The first small change I recommend is *eat less fat!* That's all you have to do to start. Learn the simple formula later in this book, follow it for two weeks or more, and if you change nothing else in your life, you'll begin to notice a little less tightness in the waist of your skirts and slacks. Doesn't that feel good? Don't you take pride in it? Won't it encourage you to take another small step—like finding a reason to walk for twenty minutes at least every other day?

You don't need our encouragement to change your life. You only need your own reason, and our job is to help you find it.

When one of my customers arrived at my salon one day feeling unattractive and depressed because of her weight problem, I shared the low-fat gospel with her. Within a short time, she grew as enthusiastic about it as I was. Maybe even more, because while I tend to be shy, she certainly isn't. I fed off her enthusiasm, she fed off mine, and eventually we became entrepreneurs. Now hundreds of people attend our seminars, thousands swear by our low-fat food products, and millions read about us and see us on network TV.

Her name, of course, is Barb Nicoll.

CHAPTER FOUR

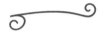

Barb's Story:
What Does It Mean When Your Dress Size Almost Equals Your Age?

Whenever I think of the pressures that many people face about losing weight and improving their health, I think about my father when I was a child.

My father was in his mid-thirties when I came along. He already had two sons, aged ten and fourteen. Boys that age are more than enough for any parent to handle. Besides, my father operated a construction company and, almost from the day my brothers, Chris and Gary, were old enough to wear hard hats, they went to work in the family business.

Running a small construction company is hard work, believe me. You put up with the stress of being a manager and the manual labor of being a tradesman. My father was gone from the house by 7:30 in the morning and didn't return until at least 6:30 each night, bringing many of his job's worries and concerns home with him. He had a set routine: Eat a huge dinner (lots of meat and gravy), lie on the sofa to watch television, maybe snack on chips and nuts, and finally fall asleep until it was time for bed. It was a routine he followed even on weekends, when he usually managed to avoid doing anything related to the business.

Dad was overweight and under a good deal of stress all the time. We never took a family vacation and, except for Christmas, we never shared much as a family. I don't recall either of my parents, for example, ever going out for a walk just to enjoy the exercise together.

If this sounds like a lot of other families you know—maybe your own—well, there's a point to be made here. My father and most people of his generation were caught up in a style of life that never gave much thought to caring for their bodies through diet and exercise. He believed the work you performed was the most important aspect of your life. Everything else—including finding leisure time to spend with your family, or hobbies to help you relax—interfered with the time you could devote to working for a living.

Life was simple: If you worked hard, you could eat well; if you ate well, you had the energy to work hard. And so it went.

Sound familiar?

Perhaps your family was like that. Many of we Late-Boomers experienced these values, and it has become difficult to deal with them in our adult lives. It doesn't make sense to blame our parents, because most of them did the best they could. I know my father felt he was doing what was best for himself and his family, and he may be surprised to read in these pages that I look back at that part of my life and his years of hard work and sacrifice with sadness. But I do.

By the time I was nine years old, my brothers had moved out of the house, leaving "me and Mom." That's how I think of my childhood—my mother, with her nice figure, usually in the kitchen cooking up a hearty meal for my father, and me, learning an appreciation for hard work and developing a taste for almost anything cooked with butter, lard, shortening and slabs of red meat.

Compared with the pain and suffering Wendy went through in her younger years, I was fortunate. I don't recall suffering pain from childhood diseases or injuries, except the usual ones, like chicken pox and measles. I took part in competitive swimming events and enjoyed horseback riding. At thirteen, I began working weekends at an upscale restaurant, clearing tables and carrying heaps of dirty dishes into the kitchen, and from there I would pick up a few more hours' work as an usher at the Shaw Festival Theatre.

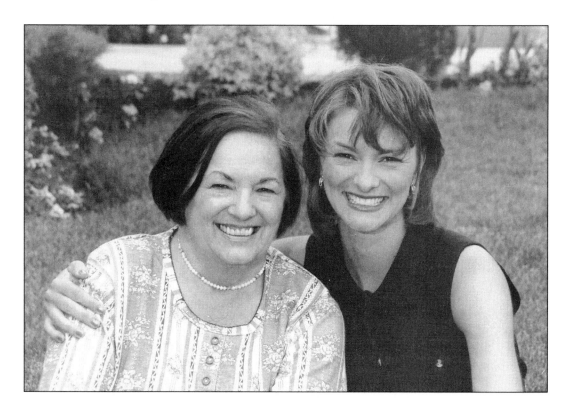

Me and my mother. Aren't the smiles similar?

By working so hard at such a young age, I was following a family tradition. Since Chris and Gary had started working in the family business at age fourteen and seventeen respectively, none of us had much of a childhood—if "childhood" means having both the freedom and the opportunity to do plenty of nothing except be a kid.

And that's the point of my reliving the past for you here. Many things we've learned about food and lifestyle in the past decade have changed both the way we raise our children and, ultimately, the world they and their children will inherit. I suppose my parents and their friends knew about the dangers of smoking, high fat content, eating too much meat and not getting enough exercise. But the knowledge didn't run deeply enough, or the dangers weren't spelled out clearly enough, for them to change their lives.

If you're over thirty, think for a moment about how much things have changed since you were a youngster, watching grown-ups and learning their values.

When you were a child, adults could stroll through a department store or grocery store smoking a cigarette, a pipe or a cigar, and few people gave it a second thought.

Chain-smokers could sit at their desks all day long, and the fumes from their cigarettes drifted throughout the building, unfiltered and unchallenged.

And until the 1980s, anyone who strapped on a pair of athletic shoes and set out trotting through the city streets was assumed to be: (a) an Olympic athlete in training; (b) a really weird person; or (c) a purse-snatcher.

So, while many of us may think we have a long way to go before becoming a healthy society, it's worth looking back to see how far we have come in our approach to food, fat and fitness. We should take encouragement from that.

When I finished high school, my father and my mother launched a bakery operation called "Mr. Meat Pie." I was expected to manage the bakery, working almost twelve hours a day, six days a week.

All day long, my parents and I dealt with the needs of the business. All evening long, and on Sundays as well, we discussed the business. After two years of that routine, I knew two things for sure: I wanted to get married and control my own life; and I expected to work hard for whatever I wanted to achieve.

Well, the marriage lasted six weeks. But the idea of working hard to reach a goal is still with me.

I needed that, because six months after my marriage collapsed, my parents closed their business. At nineteen I had no family structure, no place to live, no car or furniture, and no way of earning a living.

Fortunately, that was the end of my bad luck. (Hey, this isn't a tragedy here—it's just one woman's life and how she learned something that she wants to share with other people. So put away your hankies.)

Soon afterwards I met my future husband, Brian, and we began a relationship which led to marriage (we eloped to Las Vegas), security, and eventually a beautiful baby boy. When I became pregnant at age twenty-nine, I felt like the happiest, most excited woman in the world. I went out and bought a whole wardrobe of maternity clothes, then started wearing them right away. Holy smokes, I was only six weeks pregnant! But I couldn't wait—I wanted the world to know I was going to become a mother.

Now the next bit is going to seem a little weird to you, and some may think it's even a bit of an excuse for what happened. But it's really true.

I *loved* wearing my maternity clothes. Call it a need for identity or wild anticipation, I don't know what it was. Every morning I would get up and carefully choose the maternity dress or outfit I would wear that day. The problem, of course, was that I couldn't fill it yet. I *swam* in the things! I felt fulfilled—*Look at me! I'm going to be a mother!*—and a little silly at the same time. The baby wasn't growing fast enough to fill up all that space inside my maternity dress.

So I decided to help—by eating.

You've heard of pregnant women eating for two? I started eating for three or four. All that space was going to waste inside my maternity clothes—why not fill it up with foods I'd always loved, like donuts and milkshakes? I was soon downing two shakes a day (all that calcium in the milk had to be good for the baby, right?) and I never met a french fry I didn't like. Naturally, I cut back on my exercising as well. Why risk harming the baby by raising my pulse and breathing levels? Both of us were comfortable as could be, laying back on the sofa and watching soap operas.

When I became pregnant I weighed 125 pounds; when I entered the delivery room, I was over 200 pounds. Fill out my maternity clothes? Hey, I split the seams! My doctor, bless his heart, kept warning me about my weight. But I figured, with the baby gone, I'd soon be back to the slim old me, no sweat.

My beautiful baby boy, Jake, arrived at a hefty 9 pounds, 7 ounces. That night, lying in my hospital bed while my new baby spent his first night in the nursery, I finally worked up enough courage to pull back the sheets and examine the state of my body, now that Jake had vacated the premises. Just one little peek. Just lift the sheet, look down, and . . .

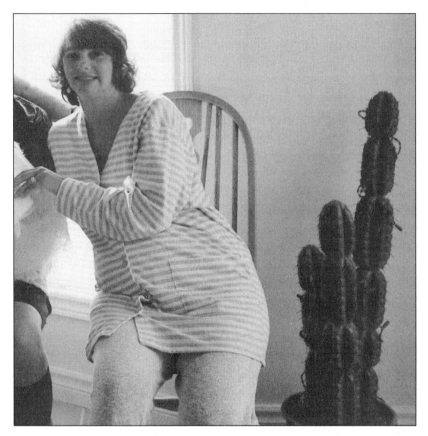

This was taken a few weeks after my son's birth. I can't blame my shape on my pregnancy, although I'd love to! It had more to do with consuming too many milkshakes and watching too much TV.

EEEEEEEEK!

Somebody had attached a strange body to my head! How could they do that? What happened to my old body, the slim, lithe torso with the smooth, flat skin? Somebody must have stolen it! Who's got it now, Sharon Stone or one of those other Hollywood hussies? And where'd I get the one I'm looking at—the one with rolls and rolls of *fat*?

When morning came, I faced the truth. Pregnancy and milkshakes had done me in. All right, I'll just have to work it off with exercise, I told myself. Really? Stumbling to a basinette at two o'clock in the morning, stubbing your toe on the dresser and tripping over your husband's shoes is not very effective in working off nine months' accumulation of fat. I simply had no time and no energy to exercise.

By the time Jake was five months old, I was still 60 pounds overweight. I collapsed into naps at least twice a day, and wore nothing but my old maternity clothes. Why not? They still fit!

That Christmas, Brian and I were invited to the usual round of parties with friends and business associates. I've always enjoyed dressing up for Christmas social events. It used to give me an opportunity to show off my figure in new outfits. But this Christmas was different. The only "new outfits" I planned to wear would be size 20 dresses borrowed from my mother. In desperation to fit back into my own clothes, I even borrowed one of my mother's classic girdles to squeeze things in place. *Arggghhh!* It was like having a long date with a boa constrictor! I walked like a wooden soldier and my voice rose half an octave. But I wore it— even after the night I arrived home from one party and was actually sick to my stomach from the pressure the girdle had been applying on my stomach all night long.

I hated that girdle. But not as much as I hated thin women.

What right did they have to look as good as I had last year at this time? What was so terrific about being anorexic? *And why did they all seem to be making eyes at my husband?!*

Oh, I was a joy to be around that Christmas.

January was even worse. I was trapped in the house by rotten weather—just me, my beautiful baby boy and my ugly three chins. I tried going for walks, but I started imagining people laughing at me and pointing, saying things like: "See that fat woman with the baby carriage? She used to be so *slim!*" My clothes were too tight, my weight kept ballooning, and my self-esteem was so low I couldn't bend over to pick it up.

Fortunately, my hair was a mess.

So I made an appointment to have it styled by my favorite hairdresser, Wendy Buckland. Wendy performed such miracles on my hair that I felt terrific—for about two days.

I returned a week later. "Make it blonde!" I told Wendy. "Blondes have more fun, right?" What I really wanted to hear was: "Yeah, and they get skinnier too!"

Being blonde made me feel better for almost a week. Then I needed another hit of hair styling.

"Let's get it permed!" I said when I arrived at Wendy's salon. Wendy, bless her heart, answered, "No!" Then she swung me around in the chair, looked me in the eye and said: "What the heck is wrong with you?"

So explained that I was fat, out of shape, depressed and tired all the time. Plus I felt worthless, useless, unattractive and a failure.

"Is that all?" Wendy replied. (She has a great sense of humor.)

Then she gave me the strangest bit of advice I'd ever heard. "Stop at a supermarket on the way home and buy a box of Fruit Loops," she said. I reminded her that Jake was still a little too young to be eating cereal. "It's not for him, silly," she said. "It's for *you*." She promised to call at six o'clock that evening. The Fruit Loops, while high in sugar content, contained almost no fat. Eating them would satisfy my appetite and help me avoid fats.

I'll admit I was a little skeptical at first. Then I figured, "What the heck. I trust this woman with my hair; might as well trust her with the rest of my body."

That evening she called and explained the concept of eliminating fat from my diet and adding muscle to my frame. The following day we went shopping together, and Wendy explained how to read the fat content on package labels, how to spot high fat where I expected to find none at all, how to replace fat in my recipes, and how to eat low-fat meals without missing a thing—except the fat.

I was hooked! I returned home with ten bags of groceries, swept half the food out of my pantry because its fat content was too high, and started planning my new lifestyle.

I began by pouring two glasses of wine and sitting down with my husband Brian. I told him my plan, explained Wendy's philosophy, and asked for his support.

When he agreed wholeheartedly, we were off!

The first to go was virtually all the red meat in our meals, replaced with turkey, chicken and fish. Having learned how to read labels for fat content, I made a game of grocery shopping. My pocket calculator accompanied me on every trip, converting fat grams to calories, then calculating the percentage of calories from fat in each product.

I didn't impose all of my new-found beliefs on Brian. He still barbecued his steak on Friday nights (and learned to cook me a wicked tuna steak!). We not only ate well, but we enjoyed our meals and looked forward to trying new low-fat recipes.

After a few weeks on the new low-fat eating schedule, I could see dramatic improvements in my weight, yet I never felt hungry or undernourished. Finally it was time to launch an activity program. Walking appealed to me, but not walking through cold rainy winter days! (Finding a baby-sitter for half an hour was also a challenge.) So I danced instead—danced all those pounds away in the comfort of my own home.

I invested in a monitor for Jake's room, one that lit up when he began to cry. Next, I paid a visit to a music store for a pair of light headphones and a couple of outrageous dance CDs, followed by a stop at an athletic store for some well-cushioned shoes and a water bottle. And Presto! I became a dance star in my own living room!

Over the next few weeks, wearing my T-shirt, shorts and headphones and, with a heavy dance beat filling my head, keeping one eye on a soap opera and the other on Jake's monitor, I boogied the pounds off. No baby-sitter, no fear of catching cold in a February blizzard, and no self-consciousness while I made up some pretty incredible moves to the dance beat! Almost before I knew it, the combination of low-fat foods and high-energy dancing chased 35 pounds off my body. Each pound I lost was another incentive to keep going, try new dance steps, add a few stretches and jumping jacks to the beat, and really build up a pleasurable sweat.

A small word of warning: If you try this method of shedding weight—and I hope you will—make sure all your valuable china, crystal and assorted fragile family heirlooms are nailed down or set safely on the floor. Otherwise, you may lose more than body weight.

Three months later, I reached my thirtieth birthday. To many women this can be a traumatic event—or so I'm told. I entered my thirties feeling more confident and upbeat than I had ever felt before. My husband and I celebrated my birthday with a weekend getaway to a hotel that just happened to have outstanding fitness facilities. We shared champagne and workouts in the gym, and had a wonderful time.

Back home, spring had arrived and I was ready to take my program on the road. Actually, it was the local high-school running track. At least twice a week we would all set off for it together: Me in my track suit, Jake in his stroller, and our dog Hogan on a leash. The next hour or so was spent with me running circuits on the track, Jake in the middle trying to follow his mother, who was running circles around him, and Hogan chewing on a bone I'd brought to keep him busy. (Dogs tend to get bored very easily by fitness workouts.)

Okay, it all sounds easy and perfect, right? The young mother who grows determined to let nothing stand in the way of regaining her youthful figure and improving her health, all while bonding to both her understanding husband and her perfect child. (Let's leave Hogan out of this for a minute.)

Well, I'm not going to lie to you anywhere in this book—including here.

Some days it was agony, especially at the beginning. I'll swear there were times when even my hair ached! (Wendy says she's the hair expert and it's impossible for your hair to ache, but I was there and she wasn't.) But the agony wasn't really necessary. If I'd prepared my body for this kind of exercise and worked up to it slowly instead of impatiently jumping into it feet-first (so to speak), it would have been much easier to take. So you needn't put up with the same level of pain as I did.

Even my bladder complained. How does a bladder let you know it's unhappy? Guess. It always happened in the middle of a workout, so I did a lot of extra laundry in those early days.

What made me stick with it? My husband thinks it's because I can be so darned stubborn at times, but there was more to it than that.

It was the payoff I got. One hour of exercise a day made me feel absolutely terrific for the other twenty-three hours. That's a super return on your investment, if you want to look at things that way. The more weight I lost and the more firm my body felt, the more inspiration I drew from it. Hey, I kept telling myself—there is nothing you cannot do!

Then Oprah Winfrey had to go and run a marathon . . .

"Well," I thought when I heard about it, "if she can do it, so can I." I may never forgive her.

See, this one's really me—the other picture of me, the one taken just after Jake's birth, was some other person. (I wish!) Anyway, this is the body I have now—and it's the one I'm going to keep!

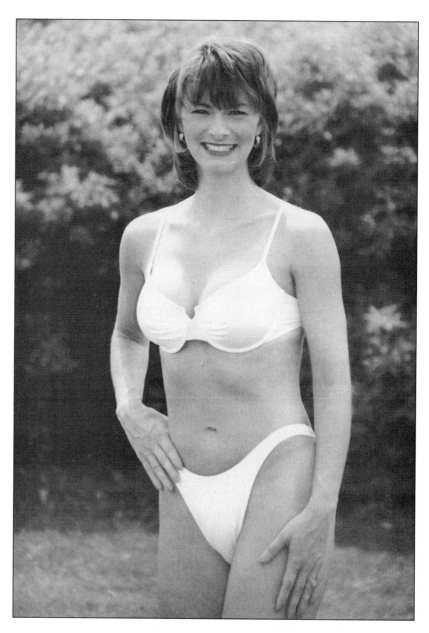

By the end of May, I entered a 3-mile (5-km) race through town. In spite of lying awake the night before the race, staring at the ceiling and asking *What have I done?!* over and over, I not only finished in twenty-one minutes, but actually won my age division!

When they called me to the podium to receive my medal, I went with Jake in my arms and tears in my eyes. I thanked my husband, who had followed my progress in the car with Jake, cheering me on by beeping the horn, and I especially thanked Wendy, who deserved the medal as much as I did.

I entered other fitness events that summer, but my eye was on a marathon scheduled for Erie, Pennsylvania, in September. So I started training for it. I would rise early in the morning, go for my run, return home just as Brian and Jake were waking up, and share breakfast with them. I found ways to maintain both my training schedule and my obligations to my husband and son. The training provided me with extra energy to go for walks in the park each evening with Brian and Jake, and still look forward to my morning run. But I kept my eye on the marathon.

About two months before the actual race, the organizers held a half-marathon to be run along the same route. We were stretched for funds at the time, but Brian borrowed a friend's tent, and a portable propane barbecue, we cleared out our bank account, and we set off on a Saturday with about seventy dollars—of which twenty-five was earmarked for my entry fee.

I should mention here that about the only thing we had never done as a family was go camping. Depending on your camping experience and your sense of humor, the next part will be either horrifying or hilarious to you.

First, we were using a borrowed tent. Borrowing someone else's tent when you have never camped before is like borrowing someone else's dog and expecting it to obey your commands. Next, we discovered that the camp site we had chosen was a dump— literally. We managed to get the tent set up on one of the few clear spaces in the area, which happened to be a flat rock. Flat rocks, of course, are cold and hard, which is not the best surface for sleeping.

That's when I discovered that I'd forgotten to pack blankets.

Naturally, it rained. That wasn't so bad, because the sound of the rain pelting on the tent managed to drown out some of the noise from a teenagers' party at the camp site next to us. The teenagers sported equal quantities of ugly tattoos, beer bottles and bad attitudes. When their party managed to finally die down, the skunks felt it was safe to come out and inspect the damage, and two of them circled our tent for the rest of the night, held at bay, I suspect, by Jake's cries—none of the above encourages a ten-month-old baby to sleep.

I honestly believe I had a total of about one hour's sleep that night, but at six o'clock in the morning I was up and ready to run. The following few hours were the longest day of my life, but I finished the half-marathon, prepared to run the full distance along the same route eight weeks later.

On the day of the marathon, Wendy and her partner, Bill, came to Erie with Brian and me. They drove along the route with me, cheering me on, and even running by my side for encouragement. Brian ran from mile 20 to mile 23 with me, and Wendy actually finished the race, running at my side into the stadium.

That final lap inside a crowded stadium with the crowd cheering us on and my friend at my side was very emotional for me. Just a year earlier, I was too depressed and too overweight to even walk around the block. Now here I was running in front of thousands of people, the end of a grueling 26-mile (42-km) course.

I was awarded another medal for my achievement, and each time I hold it in my hand it reminds me of how far I have come and how much I have benefited from the love and support of my family and friends.

If I could come so far so fast—changing from an overweight woman ashamed to be seen in public to a marathon medal-winner running in her shorts and T-shirt—Wendy and I must be on to something. We might be unique—everyone is, in various ways—but we didn't consider ourselves exceptional. If we needed to learn how to shop for and prepare low-fat meals, other people must as well. If we could find activities we enjoyed, instead of looking at exercise as a form of self-torture, maybe we could help other people find them. If we could eliminate pain and reduce the effects of diseases that doctors keep telling us are incurable—like Wendy's arthritis—through diet and exercise, maybe we could help others do it too.

We began by placing a small advertisement in our local news-

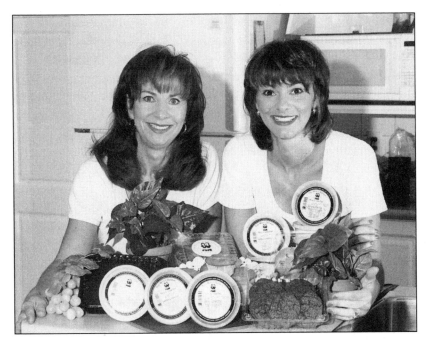

We have our own line of food products, now sold in hundreds of stores across North America. Who says you need high fat content to make great-tasting dips, brownies and muffins?

paper, promoting seminars titled "Eat Low-Fat and Get Fit!" We charged $35 admission, bought food samples to share with those who attended the seminars, and added optional shopping trips to local supermarkets at $10 person.

It was like releasing water from behind a dam. From our first seminar, the momentum built up. I began calling the various media—newspapers, radio and TV stations, anyone who would get out the word—and we were invited as guests to talk about our approach to diet and wellness.

Often, during our shopping-trip lessons, people would say things like, "Why can't they make a low-fat dip?" or "Do you think anybody will ever come up with a low-fat chocolate cookie?"

Well, no one else seemed to be in a hurry to do it, so Wendy and I did it. We developed the recipes, chose quality food producers to make them for us, and camped out in front of supermarket buyers' offices until they agreed to carry our products. We gave free samples in stores carrying our products, developed promotion materials like posters and photographs, and frankly worked our butts off to turn something we believed in into something that could benefit others as much as it had benefited us.

Had someone suggested a year and a half earlier that I might become a poster girl for a low-fat and fitness, I would have held my stomach laughing . . . if I could have gotten my arms around the darn thing!

Now we have a company, a business plan, new careers and a book.

And it all started with a box of Fruit Loops.

I'm not pretending that all of this was as easy as it may sound. But nothing worthwhile is ever easy. Anything we do easily has little value to us. It's the things we work at—getting an education, raising a child, holding a relationship together—that we value most.

My goal is to encourage you to realize two things.

First, don't ever assume that any goal is unattainable. I don't consider myself exceptional—blessed, perhaps, with basic good health and support from people who care about me—but not outstanding in terms of athletic ability or determination. Remember that I'm the same person who lay on a sofa devouring milkshakes, donuts and french fries, waiting for my baby to arrive. So I share the same weaknesses with everyone else.

Second, I can't emphasize the importance of support. In my case, it was the encouragement of Wendy and my husband, and they made all the difference to me.

The real lesson here? Find someone who will encourage you in your efforts . . . who believes in your ability to reach your goal . . . and who understands it will be difficult at times and that you may stumble, but who never gives up and never lets *you* give up.

I know many of you who read this will be single parents, pressed by demands of time and money to just make it through each day. I was fortunate enough to have a partner whom I could lean on both emotionally and economically, and the challenges you face may make my achievements look almost easy.

There is nothing I can do except present myself as one example of what can be accomplished through finding inner strength. I honestly believe we all have that strength within us. Some of us may

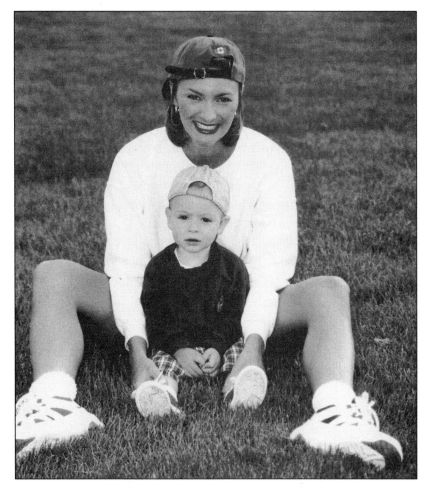

Taking a break with Jake during one of our workouts. Mine consists of jogging a few laps around the track; Jake's job is to inspect dandelions.

have hidden it away from domineering parents or spouses. Or it has been weakened by combating other challenges in our lives.

But if you're reading this book, you must have some plan or dream to improve your appearance and wellness. I suggest you hold onto it and use whatever strength you can find to make it come true.

Wendy, who is a much stronger advocate of weight lifting than I (I think of running marathons the same way Wendy thinks of bench-pressing her weight), has always bragged that the more you use your muscles, the stronger they become. So what seems to be impossible today can seem ridiculously easy in a few months.

I think inner strength works the same way. If you had just enough strength to invest time and money in reading this book, you have enough to take the next step—cutting excess fat in your diet. And when you do that, you'll have built up the strength to start an activity program—long walks, dancing in your living room, lifting cans of tomatoes as weights, or whatever it takes.

Please take even the smallest strength and work up from there.

When you make enough progress to see how low-fat eating and fitness activity have literally changed your life, write us and tell us your story. We're already planning another book, featuring tales of people who have managed to turn dreams into reality.

We'll refer to them all as "heroes," because that's what they'll be to us.

So make yourself a hero (if you think that's just a sandwich, remember to hold the butter and mayo!), and tell me about it. Okay?

CHAPTER FIVE

The Fat You Eat Is the Fat You Wear

When we hold seminars on low-fat eating, or appear on television shows talking about becoming *Armed and Dangerous*, people often comment about our demeanor. "You two seem to enjoy what you do so much!" they tell us. "Are you always so bubbly and optimistic?"

No, not always. But we enjoy most aspects of our lives most hours of the day. We think you can as well. The whole idea behind this book is to arm you with the means and the ways to face the darker sides of life that we encounter from time to time. After all, you don't put on happiness like it's a new spring coat. True happiness and contentment are part of your being, every bit as much as the rest of you—body and soul.

It's not snacking—it's "grazing."

Sometimes our bodies just won't cooperate. There we are, eating three low-fat, healthy meals a day, and we still get peckish with a couple of hours to go until dinner. This used to be called snacking, which suggests potato chips, peanuts, cookies and candy. If you're sincerely trying to lose weight, these goodies have as much guilt as calories. So don't call it snacking.

Call it grazing. And make the foods healthy, satisfying and low-fat.
Naturally, this suggests standbys like fruit, carrot sticks and celery stalks.
Good, but boring. Here are some different suggestions:

★ Crusty French bread with homemade preserves or our no-fat bruschetta

★ Microwaved potato with salsa and non-fat sour cream

★ Pretzels, rice cakes and non-fat frozen yogurt

★ Roasted turkey breast cut in small portions; top each with a slice of Vadalia onion

★ Chick-peas, washed and drained, with a small amount of salt (skip the salt if you're watching your sodium intake)

★ Baked potato chips—look for those with 10 percent or fewer calories from fat

Like it or not, the roots of self-esteem and self-confidence are deeply embedded in the way we look and the state of our health. *And both of these are directly affected by the amount of fat in our diet and the level of physical exercise in our life.*
We'll deal with the health question first.

If you are in a state of good physical health, you already possess a basic reason to be happy . . . and the older you are, the more happiness you can derive from that fact. All the riches you can acquire in the world, and all the fame and flattery you can buy or borrow, cannot soften the impact of a doctor staring back at you over her glasses and telling you that your disease is terminal. Believe it.

We already know the basics of good health. They involve genes, nutrition and exercise. Score high on all three, don't tempt fate, and maybe we'll be there to light the candles on your ninetieth-birthday cake. And if your gene selection wasn't as good as it might be, that's all the more reason to change the things you can, isn't it?

"So what else is new?" you may be asking by now. "Lose weight and stay active? I've been hearing that for years."

To which we might reply: "So how come you're still overweight and crushing a sofa cushion?" But we won't....

What's new is this:

First, those of us who challenged the dangers of nicotine and watched society turn on the tobacco companies with a vengeance are now shifting our attention to the effects of excess fats in our foods. They're not as immediately obvious as tobacco smoke, perhaps. But the effects are just as deadly. In our opinion, we are all on the crest of a rising wave of awareness about excessive fat in our food. When it builds full momentum and finally reaches the shore, the wave will wash over us, with a cleansing effect on food processors and producers. It's up to all of us to keep the wave moving and reduce unnecessary fats. We can start by alerting large segments of the population to their effects.

Next, we think people are growing more realistic and sophisticated about achieving and maintaining a healthy lifestyle. All social changes begin on the fringes. From macrobiotics in the 1960s to the jogging craze of the 1970s through the introduction of expensive (and often unnecessary) home gyms in the 1980s, the concept of wellness has slowly crept into our collective consciousness. It has been made stronger, we think, by changing roles in our society as well. A generation or two ago, grandmothers were pictured wearing high-button shoes, small glasses and funny flowered hats—women whose sexual activity faded around the time menopause arrived. Well, forget that. Sexuality is what you make it, and if you're still making it in your sixties and beyond, go for it. Of course, going for it is one thing; getting "it" is another, and that's where your good health and appearance come in, right?

Which leads us to the final point:

Among the most dramatic and least-surprising medical discoveries of the last decade was the announcement that people who enjoy a positive mental outlook tend to enjoy good physical health.

Think about that for a moment.

Maybe you've been ignoring all the healthy reasons to cut fat from your diet, losing weight and toning up your muscles in the process. Why? Because all those authority figures keep saying "It's good for you!" Which is reason enough not to do it. (Sometimes we think the strongest voice inside us is thirteen years old, still convinced that all the wisdom of the world resides in the pockets of its jeans and the tracks of its record collection....)

We're not authority figures. (Just ask our kids.) We're your friends. So we say:

Do it for "superficial" reasons.

★ Do it because it will make you look more attractive and let you choose your clothes from a wider wardrobe.

★ Do it because it will draw more attention from your partner, and perhaps more appreciative glances from people you might consider as a partner.

★ Do it because it will improve your sex life, pleasure-seeking hussy that you are.

★ Do it because it will make your friends jealous, envious or maybe even pleased for you.

★ Do it because, in a complex world where we are so often removed from the end results of our occupations, you will be the 100 percent beneficiary of your efforts—and not many things in life offer so direct a reward.

★ Finally, do it because, by feeling better about yourself and opening new opportunities for happiness, you will without doubt improve at least your chances of becoming healthier and more disease-resistant. And who can argue with that?

> *Eat one large bucket of theater popcorn made with coconut oil, and you are ingesting the same amount of saturated fat you would consume by eating bacon and eggs for breakfast, a Big Mac and fries for lunch and steak with sour cream for dinner every day for four days.*[1]

---

[1] *Bulletin*: Center for Science in the Public Interest (Washington, DC: 1994).

Fat's in the funniest places (Ha, Ha).

For most of us, eating low-fat sounds relatively easy. We asked some friends to name the foods they would cut back to reduce their fat intake. Then we asked them to name the foods they would eat to replace those foods.

Here are the ones they mentioned most often to reduce their fat consumption:

- Bacon
- Potato chips and fast snacks
- Fish and chips, fried chicken, other fried foods
- Ice cream
- Buttered popcorn, butter generally
- Sour cream on baked potatoes
- French fries
- Pastries—cakes, pies, etc.

Fairly predictable, right?

Interestingly, nobody mentioned things such as condiments. You like mayonnaise on your sandwich? Virtually every prepared mayonnaise is 100 percent fat! Think you'll switch to so-called Lite mayonnaise? That's nice. The most popular brand of Lite mayonnaise is only 90 percent fat. "But how much harm can a spoonful of mayo do to me?" you may be asking. Okay, put a 1-ounce (28 g) spoonful of mayo on your sandwich every other day of the year. Congratulations—at the end of one year you have ingested almost 10 pounds (4.5 kg) of pure fat! Not just calories—fat that your body will hoard away in secret and not-so-secret places.

 ere are some other foods that no one mentioned cutting back on to reduce their fat intake, along with the typical levels of fat they contain as a percentage of total calories:

★ Bologna (beef and pork)   80 + percent

★ Cheese (packaged Cheddar)   70 + percent

★ Crackers   30–45 percent

★ Eggs   65 percent

★ Hot dog wieners   80 + percent

What foods would they eat to replace the ones they cut from their diets?

★ Salads (with dressing)

★ Fish—especially tuna and salmon

★ Nuts and fruit

★ Lean meats

It's a short list, but it sounds healthy—until you examine things a little more closely.

Consider the esteemed salad—lettuce, tomato, celery, a little onion, some sweet pepper perhaps—not an ounce of fat to be found. Until someone lathers it with dressing. Okay, a salad without dressing doesn't turn too many cranks for people. But if "salad dressing" means oil and vinegar, you're adding another ounce or two of 100 percent fat from the oil.

Fish is fine. Broiled and lightly spiced with a splash of lemon juice is very nice. But fish are like people—too many of them are swimming around with more fat than needed. (The fish need the fat—we don't.) Many brands of canned salmon derive 50 percent or more of their calories from fat that occurs naturally in the fish. Broiled or baked Atlantic salmon is delicious; it's also about 35 percent fat. Tuna has less fat—about 30 percent raw, less when canned in water. Choose tuna canned in oil and congratulations— or maybe it should be condolences—one brand of canned tuna in oil delivers a whopping 78 percent of its calories as fat. Of course, many people carefully choose tuna canned in water, which they mix with a healthy dollop of mayo to make tuna-salad sandwiches, all the while telling themselves they're cutting back on fat. You don't do that, do you? Good.

Nuts and fruit are undoubtedly healthy, but be aware: almost all nuts contain 75 percent or more oil as measured against their calories. Pecans score very high in fat content—as much as 90 percent. Scoop an ounce (28 g) of fresh salted pecans in your mouth and expect to discover 21 grams of fresh fat somewhere on your body soon.

Fruits are fine too. But be careful. If you enjoy avocados, you probably won't enjoy discovering that a raw California avocado scores 86 percent of its 300 + calories from fat.

Lean meats? Nice idea, but lean red meats are like calorie-reduced dressings—you're usually only fooling yourself. Extra-lean ground beef, broiled to medium, has 58 percent of its calories in the form of saturated fats; every 3 ounces (84 g) you consume delivers about 14 grams of fat to your system. In fact, virtually all red meat labeled "lean" contains between 40 and 60 percent fat levels, when measured as a percentage of calories.

Hi, It's Wendy:

Please don't become discouraged by all these statistics on fat content in your food. It's much too easy to throw up your hands and say "Everything I like to eat has too much fat in it, so what's the use?" Remember that your body still requires at least some fat each day—about 1 tablespoon (15 mL). If you eliminated 100 percent of natural fats in everything you ate, you wouldn't be able to maintain your optimum level of good health.

We included all the "bad news" about fat because it's important to "Know your enemy"—or at least know where he's hiding. When you're aware of certain places that are full of danger, your common sense tells you not to go in there without evaluating the risk and bringing some support with you.

For example—butter and cooking oil are not really "bad guys" in the kitchen until they start ganging up on you. So just get in the habit of keeping butter and oils in their place. Here's an example:

When cooking shallots or onions, a little oil or butter—never more than a teaspoon or two—is needed to start breaking down their cellulose content. Once you're aware that you've used oil or butter this way for one meal or one place in a recipe, avoid using it in others. For example, when you use butter or oil for the onions, avoid it when preparing the rest of the meal. Sprinkle lemon juice on cooked vegetables and use a non-fat dressing on your salad.

Whatever you do, don't let the high-fat content of many foods discourage you. Just arm yourself with the information we've provided, and press on to victory.

Make friends with Three Amigos who'll help you become Armed and Dangerous: Food, Exercise and Attitude.

Reducing the fat content of your meals is the single most important step you can take to produce an honest-to-goodness visual improvement in your body. Seeing the difference that substantially lower fat consumption can make will create immediate positive reinforcement. Positive reinforcement means you won't need someone patting you on the head, saying "That's a good little girl," or hiding in the refrigerator ready to slap your hand when you reach for the butter or margarine. All the encouragement will come from within, because your own body will tell you it's feeling better.

Later, we'll cover the information you'll need to slash your fat intake without feeling the pain of deprivation. But here are the basic rules as they apply to your food:

★ Along with reducing fat content, try reducing the size of your meal portions. We all have echoes of a parent's voice telling us to eat all the food on our plate or we won't get: (a) dessert, (b) to play outside, (c) to watch television. So we tend to clean our plates, even if they hold far more food than our bodies need. Solution: invest in smaller dinner plates (don't laugh—many people discovered it made an immediate difference), or at least serve yourself smaller portions on the plates you now own.

★ Accept the fact that you may have bad days, when you simply *must* slather butter and mayo on your next sandwich.

Just vow to get back on track the next day. Don't beat up on yourself for sliding a little—it's a waste of time and doesn't help your self-esteem.

★ Organize your food purchases at the supermarket. Then, at home, you're always surrounded with healthy options. (Chapter 8 covers the supermarket scene in detail.)

★ An oldie hint, but still a goodie: Shop for your groceries immediately after a meal. You'll spend less, and make fewer impulse purchases of foods you don't need.

★ Don't let the rest of the world dictate your healthy choices. When choosing a restaurant, call ahead to ask about their low-fat menu selections. (The better restaurants are already shifting in this direction and they'll appreciate your interest; if the restaurant seems annoyed or amused by your question regarding low-fat selections, maybe they're not one of the better restaurants, *n'est-ce pas?*)

★ When traveling, take responsibility for your own diet. On long car trips, pack low-fat sandwiches and snacks— you'll not only avoid the high-fat content of the offerings at many fast-food outlets, but you'll also save time and money on your travels. If traveling by air, request a special dietary meal and you may enjoy a bonus: On many airlines, the low-fat meals are frankly more interesting than those served to regular passengers.

What's all this stuff about a "set point" anyway?

Many people who try to lose weight through calorie-reduced diets succeed for a while. Then they watch their weight climb back to where it was before they began. This makes them feel very good about themselves.

"That's my set point," they say smugly—usually while patting their tummies. "That's where my body likes to be."

This is a very interesting theory. It's based on the idea that our bodies are dumb enough to *want* to be overweight, to *want* to

Fat's in the Funniest Places (Cont'd)
Percentage of calories from fat in typical foods:[2]

Cracklin' Bran breakfast cereal	33 percent
Frozen broccoli in creamy Italian sauce	60 percent
Sesame bagel chips	62 percent
Yogurt-covered peanuts	65 percent
Granular black caviar	68 percent
Durkee shredded coconut	91 percent
Canned/marinated artichoke hearts	100 percent
Coffee creamer	100 percent

carry all that extra weight around, putting a strain on the heart, the liver and several other essential parts. It's like having an unruly child who "wants" to stay up until three o'clock in the morning playing video games so, after failing to discipline him, you just shrug your shoulders and say: "That's what he *wants* to do." People who buy this "set point" story are saying: "My body wants to be fat, so I guess I'll just let it do what it wants to do."

Your body wants to be fat? How fat was it when you were in your teen years or your twenties? What was its "set point" then? We'll bet it was much lower. Which proves that a set point can be changed. Unfortunately, in the case of most people in their forties, it has changed by moving up.

If our bodies can move their set points up, we can help nudge them down. It takes a little effort—but anyone who thinks that fitness and weight loss come out of a bottle is reading the wrong book. We said we'd make this as much fun and as little effort as possible, but it ain't all easy.

A road map for your cruise control.

Who was that terrible socialite who said, "You can never be too rich or too thin"? Now there's a snob for you. Of course you can be too thin! We don't advocate organized anorexia here. A library

---

[2]Karen Bellerson's *The Complete and Up-to-Date Fat Book*, (Garden City Park, NY: Avery, 1993).

of information exists to guide us toward the ideal weight and height combination, based on years of research and data. So forget about "never being too thin." (On the other hand, we could be persuaded to accept her economic theory . . . .)

Below is a weight chart that's worth following in setting a target for you to hit. Instead of asking you to decide if you are small-boned, medium-boned or big-boned, we chose one based on age groups. Let's be realistic: lowering your weight after age forty is twice as hard as it was at age twenty. So age cannot be overlooked.

The weight guide includes both men and women. Generally, choose the lower portion of the range if you're a woman. For example, if you're over age 35 and 5 feet, 5 inches tall, the weight range is 126–162 pounds. That's a difference of 36 pounds. If you're a woman, divide the difference by 2 (= 18 pounds) and add to the low weight, giving you a target range of 126–144 pounds. For men, subtract half the difference from the high weight (162 − 18 = 144) for a range of 144–162 pounds.

HEIGHT	WEIGHT BY AGE	
	19 to 34	35 and over
5'0"	97–128	108–138
5'1"	101–132	111–143
5'2"	104–137	115–148
5'3"	107–141	119–152
5'4"	111–146	122–157
5'5"	114–150	126–162
5'6"	118–155	130–167
5'7"	121–160	134–172
5'8"	125–164	138–178
5'9"	129–169	142–183
5'10"	132–174	146–188
5'11"	136–179	151–194
6'0"	140–184	155–199

SOURCE: 1994 Health Bulletin, U.S. Department of Agriculture/Department of Health and Human Services.

We deserve a break every day—from FAT!

McDonald's, the fast-food chain who built a market for adults with its "You deserve a break today!" theme in the 1980s, has announced a new burger aimed exclusively at the adult market. Called "Arch Deluxe," the new menu item from the Golden Arches has a potato flour bun, seasoned hamburger meat, stone-ground mustard, mayonnaise and optional bacon. "This is another big step down the wrong road," said Michael Jacobson of the Center for Science in the Public Interest. "I estimate that this product at minimum will provide half a day's worth of fat, saturated fat and sodium".[3]

Perform liposuction in your own home.

Right this moment, while you're sitting here reading this book, a woman somewhere in the world cringes as the suction tip of a modified Hoover vacuum cleaner is being slipped under her skin. It may be in her thighs, her buttocks, her tummy or some other part of her body. Wherever it is, the vacuum cleaner is about to start sucking fat cells out from beneath her skin while she visualizes herself as a slim attractive beauty—the girl she once was and so desperately wants to be again.

We don't wish to humiliate this poor woman, and the thousands of others who will probably receive the same treatment today. Nor do we want to disparage the doctors and nurses performing the treatment—they're undoubtedly skilled, dedicated professionals who care about their patients' well-being.

But it's all so unnecessary![4]

First, the results are never as satisfying as the women hope they will be. You can't mess with your body this way, no matter

---

[3] Associated Press News Service, May 8, 1996.

[4] We're talking about shaping your entire body this way. If you honestly try to reduce one area of your body through physical activity and low-fat diet, and it still doesn't work, then liposuction may be a reasonable alternative. But we suspect it's used, not as a last resort, but as an easy "out" for people who haven't read this book.

how skilled the surgeon is, and expect not to suffer trauma of some kind. And you can't expect fat that's been comfortably ensconced beneath your skin for twenty years or so to go quietly.

Next, there is a substantial period of recovery for many women. It may be several months before they dare to wear shorts or a bathing suit. They're hiding themselves away while the skin—which is not nearly as elastic as it was in their twenties— manages to relax its folds and adhere to the muscle mass beneath it.

Finally, it ain't cheap, baby. Some women can laugh off the several thousand dollars for the procedure and recovery, plus another few grand to lie around a luxury spa out of sight and relax. Good for them. But we can't believe they wouldn't rather see the money invested somewhere, even if it's in a new wardrobe or a few new gold baubles.

If you've become so distressed about your figure and the excess fat on various parts of your body that you've seriously con- sidered liposuction, we understand. For the benefit of good looks alone, we're on your side when it comes to ridding yourself of fleshy folds and thundering thighs.

But, please, at least give the food and fitness suggestions in this book a reasonable chance to show what they can do.

We don't think there is an unemployment crisis among plastic surgeons in North America. We don't even want to start one. But we think reducing fat can be accomplished more easily, more cheaply and more safely in your own kitchen and living room than in the operating room.

Check off these facts if you agree with them:

❑ I won't snack. I'll graze on filling foods without fat.

❑ Excess weight may soon be as socially unacceptable as smoking.

❑ Good physical health and good mental health are intertwined.

❑ I refuse to beat up on myself if I fail to follow my low-fat rules without fail. I'll just get back on track and keep going.

❑ I'm in charge of my own life, my own weight program and my own happiness, and nobody else will interfere.

❑ My ideal target weight is: _____ lb.
Today's date is: _____
My weight today is: _____ lb.

If you don't agree with a statement above, write your reasons here:

_____

_____

_____

_____

_____

_____

CHAPTER SIX

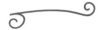

A Is for Activity

By this point, the vast majority of people we talk to during our *Armed and Dangerous* seminars are nodding their heads, smiling and saying "You're right. Too much fat's not good for us and some fats are really risky. Right on! Out with the fat and in with the good stuff!"

Then we mention exercise.

That's when a lot of people slide down into their seats, study their manicures, or go looking for the washroom.

Hey, we understand. Few of us are natural athletes, and most of us have earned the right to take things easy as much as possible.

Exercise is like anything else in life—if you don't enjoy doing it, you won't get much out of it. In our experience, the thought of starting an exercise program has turned more people off weight control and a healthy lifestyle than any other single factor.

We have an idea:

For the rest of this chapter, let's banish the word "exercise" and substitute "activity." If finding ways to become more active is easier to swallow than visualizing yourself drenched in sweat from exercise, what the heck. What's in a name, anyway?

Note from Barb:

I'm one of those people who enjoys exercising. But I'll admit that it's a little bit like enjoying sushi—some people will never get used to it. If you like aerobics or swimming or jogging, that's great! But you should read this section anyway. Perhaps your spouse, partner or friend just can't get as much from exercise as you do, and he or she will want to hear about this.

Of course, if you're already in an exercise program, stay with it—especially if it's both fun for you and beneficial for your body.

You already know that activity burns away calories. What you may not realize is the tremendous amount of activity you need to make a difference in your caloric intake. We used to trade activity for food binges—you know: "I'll have french fries with dinner, then I'll jog around the block and burn it off."

Here are the cold, hard facts:

If you weigh 150 pounds, and consume a large serving (40 pieces) of french fries, those crispy little suckers delivered 600 calories to your body—about half of them as fat—and you'd better be prepared to run—not jog, but *flat-out run*—for almost an hour to burn them off.

Most people overestimate the amount of weight they lose from strenuous activity. Everything else being equal, burning away extra weight means hard work—the kind of hard work that quickly turns many people off a wellness program.

Obviously, the answer is to stop everything from being equal. Then we can burn more calories with less activity, right?

The secret lies in changing your fat/muscle proportion, and the theory is easy to grasp.

Picture yourself riding a horse. (Stay with us on this, and please don't be offended—it's just our way of illustrating a basic fact of physiology.) Now imagine that the horse represents all the muscles in your body, and you, sitting up there in the saddle, represent ... um ... the *fat*. This is how you go through each day of your life: Your muscles do the work, and your fat content is merely along for the ride.

When your body burns calories, it doesn't do it in proportion to the fat in your body. Those calories are flamed away to support your body's muscles, through metabolism. The greater your muscle mass, the higher your metabolism; the higher your metabolism, the more calories you'll burn twenty-four hours a day. That's right—add to your muscle mass and you'll even burn more energy while you're sleeping!

Here's where weight lifting becomes especially valuable. Lifting pieces of iron and steel sounds like the worst part of the "E" word we promised not to use in this chapter. But if you're serious about fast-tracking your weight loss ... about shaping your body to make it more attractive ... about dissolving the excess fat you've accumulated over the years ... and about accelerating your metabolic rate to make it easier to *keep* it off in the future ... give the following at least some thought before you reject the idea completely.

★ *Nothing builds muscles better than resistance.*
That's all weight lifting is—resistance that your muscles must overcome.

★ *Weight lifting can be very selective.* All-round aerobics are vital for full improvement in heart and lung performance and shouldn't be ignored (although brisk walking is as effective as any activity in this regard). But weight lifting targets specific muscle groups for visible improvements, such as pectoral, thigh and arm muscles.

★ *Weight lifting won't make you look grotesque.* Many people are frankly turned off by the extremes to which some body-builders go. (And many people are turned on by the same effects, so to each her own....) If you're a woman who rejects weight lifting because you're afraid you may start looking like Arnold Schwarzenegger in drag, forget it—it won't happen unless you set that particular goal and work very hard at it for a very long time.

★ *You won't need a second mortgage on your house to get started.* Sure, you can invest several thousand dollars in a chrome-and-leather torture machine that will fill a good-sized room. But don't. One set of barbells properly used will get you started. And many fitness experts such as Covert Bailey believe free weights—barbells and so on—are actually far better than machines at building fitness because they tend to demand more work from a wider range of muscles.

★ *Every ounce of new muscle brings another benefit with it.* The psychological benefits of adding well-toned muscle to your body are extraordinary. You may not begin feeling like Wonder Woman or Superman, but you'll almost certainly walk, work, dress and live with new pride in yourself. If you're a woman, you'll enjoy discovering the joy of a smaller waist, a firmer bust and fewer things that jiggle when you walk. If you're a man, you'll find fewer occasions when it's necessary to suck in your stomach (which tends to make your face turn red and your expression pretty silly, guys) in the presence of younger women.

★ *The more muscle you have, the more fat you'll burn.* Sounds strange? Not really, when you stop to think about it. Fat is just baggage; muscle is *you*. People with a higher muscle-to-fat ratio burn off more calories *just sitting still. Or sleeping!* Here you are jogging your buns off—or trying to—and other people are burning extra calories while having a nap. We ask you—is that fair?

Weight lifting is a whole topic in itself. We suggest you consider it seriously, then do four things:

1. Discuss it with your doctor and evaluate any risk involved.

2. Obtain sufficient guidance from any of several good books on the topic—or ask for assistance from a weight-lifting friend.

3. Always perform warm-up exercises to avoid muscle damage.

4. Stay with it during the critical first few weeks until you begin noticing the visual improvement that will almost certainly keep you going.

Typical Activities—Calories Burned per Minute (by body weight)

Activity	120 lbs	150 lbs	200 lbs
Golf (foursome, cart)	3.2	3.8	6.3
Tennis (doubles)	3.4	4.0	6.5
Weight lifting (light)	4.4	5.0	7.5
Walking (17-minute mile)	4.8	5.2	7.9
Dancing (square & round)	6.4	7.0	9.5
Softball/baseball	6.6	7.2	9.7
Walking (15-minute mile)	6.6	7.2	9.7
Swimming (50 yds./minute)	8.5	9.1	11.6
Weight lifting (strenuous)	9.4	10.0	12.5
Cycling (5-minute mile)	10.0	10.6	13.1
Basketball	11.4	12.0	14.5
Skiing (cross-country)	13.4	14.0	16.5

One more conspiracy to worry about: The world doesn't want you to be active.

Sometimes it seems that the primary goal of civilized society is to turn all of us into sloths. So we ride in wood-paneled elevators with piped-in music, or on polished escalators that carry us effortlessly from one level to another. Prime parking spaces are always closest to the entrance to buildings and malls, and moving walkways transport us silently through airports—after we've just spent five hours in a cramped location that barely lets us move our necks.

Think about these activities—the kind you can perform literally every working day—and note the typical number of calories burned for each one:

★ Parking your car at the far end of the parking lot instead of near the door (20 calories)

★ Walking up five flights of stairs to your office, down at lunch, back up after lunch, and down again after work (200 calories)

★ Walking six blocks to a restaurant and back for lunch (150 calories)

★ Walking half a mile with a friend after dinner (75 calories)

We count almost 450 calories you will have burned off each day. If you're eating low-fat foods, with 20 percent or fewer calories from fat, you'll be burning off mostly body fat. At the same time, you'll be adding a little more muscle to your frame—not a heck of a lot, but every bit counts.

Five most common reasons people have for not using expensive exercise equipment:[1]

1. *Can't hear the TV while doing the exercise.*

2. *Can't do the exercise as comfortably as it appeared in the TV commercials.*

3. *Can't afford the time.*

4. *Don't have room for an exercise area in their home.*

5. *It's boring.*

Percentage growth from 1990 to 1995 of "Play It Again" retail outlets specializing in used exercise equipment:[2]
1628 percent

[1]Knight-Ridder/Tribune News Service, *Toronto Star*, April 15, 1996.
[2]*Toronto Star*, April 15, 1996.

Making a point of climbing stairs instead of standing in elevators reflects the third friend you can enlist in growing *Armed and Dangerous*: Attitude. If your attitude is positive enough, you can accomplish any realistic goal.

We really want to stress this aspect of wellness, because it is the one weapon that only you can provide. Your doctor, your supermarket and your shopping mall can all provide you with the guidance, the foods and the athletic gear you need to arm yourself against fat. Your partner, family and friends can (and should) provide you with the encouragement to achieve your goal. But none of this will work without a determination by you to start changing things in your life—even the smallest things, in the smallest ways.

Hi, It's Wendy:

When Barb and I first began planning this book, we naturally gave a lot of thought to the title. *"Lose Fat and Get Fit"* was the kind of phrase that popped into our heads. Tell it like it is. Get the message out.

As a description of our goal, it was fine. But as a message to the millions of people we wanted to reach, it flopped. Who doesn't want to lose fat? Who doesn't want to get fit? Everybody wants it, most people have tried it, and the majority have failed.

Why? Not because they were weak, or dumb or uncommitted. It had to be something else. It had to be because nothing had tapped the energy that we all have within us—the energy that a mother finds to raise the front end of a car to free her child, for example. In other words, *almost all of us can tap the energy it takes to save someone else's life, but we have a problem tapping it to save our own.*

Call it anger, call it determination, call it fear, if you want. But the energy resides within all of us. When our lives are threatened, we become as strong as we need to be to save ourselves. We become, for a time at least, *Armed and Dangerous*. Don't mess with my personal security. Don't threaten my child. Don't push me too far.

That's the strength we want to reach in all of you. If you choose to get angry at the effects of fat on your health, on your appearance, on your self-esteem and on the enjoyment you deserve from the one life you're likely to live, hooray for you! Arm yourself with the facts of fat. Make it dangerous for anything or anyone to shake your belief in yourself!

Welcome to the club, Slim.

Three things our bodies do with calories.

It helps to understand what our bodies do with the calories in our food, so without getting into a review of high-school health classes, here they are:

1. *Our bodies burn some calories as energy.* From the continuous beating of your heart to bench-pressing your weight, all the muscles in your body use energy—measured in calories—to do their work. The more work they do, the more calories you use up. Pretty basic stuff.

2. *Our bodies burn some calories as heat.* Calories are the fuel in our furnace that keeps our body temperature at a normal 98.6° Fahrenheit (37° Celsius). Now here's an interesting fact we discovered: the older we get, the less heat our bodies produce, per pound of weight. That's why on a cold winter day, when you—an intelligent, mature and responsible grown-up—are bundled in wool, leather and the odd buffalo hide, you are amazed to see children leaping around in light jackets and shirts, without mittens and hats. "Don't they know this weather is dangerous for brass monkeys?" you say to yourself with annoyance. The answer is no, they don't. For a variety of reasons, their bodies are burning more calories, elevating their temperature, and making them more comfortable than you are.

3. *Our bodies store the remaining calories as fat.* Eating fat you can't use right away is like having an oil furnace in the wintertime, and the delivery truck arrives with more oil than you need that night to stay warm. What happens to all those extra gallons of oil? It goes in the tank for later. Where's your tank? If you're a man, probably your belly. If you're a woman, start with your hips and thighs and head out from there.

Let's add one more thing to the picture.

As we get older—especially past the dreaded age forty checkpoint—our muscle mass normally begins to decrease. Yet muscles are the best calorie-burning machines in our bodies. We can increase our body heat by being more active, just like children do when they're hopping around waiting for the school bus without jackets or mittens. Muscles actually can burn up to fifty times more calories when they're at work than when they're resting.

Here's another fact to consider:

The actions of our muscles account for 90 percent of our body's use of calories. So if you eat 2,000 calories a day, you had better find a way of burning 1,800 of them through muscle action, or your oil tank is going to start overflowing into your basement.

When you eat sugar, the level of glucose (also called "blood sugar") begins to rise almost immediately. This is the "sugar rush" some people feel from eating candy. Increased levels of glucose in your blood triggers your pancreas to go to work, producing insulin. Insulin zips around, affecting every part of your body (except your brain—we've always found that interesting ...). When body cells detect insulin, they open up to admit the glucose, so your blood sugar soon drops.

Most of the glucose is being directed toward your muscle cells. But when your muscles are out of shape, they develop "insulin insensitivity." (A woman friend of ours who has been married more times than she cares to count heard this and said, "Which proves that muscles are basically male," but we think she was just being cynical.)

Insulin insensitivity prevents the muscle cells from absorbing as much glucose as they should. So unfit people walk around for a long time after eating with elevated levels of blood sugar.

Here's where the really cruel part begins.

All that glucose in the blood of unfit people gives up trying to ease its way into muscles cells that suffer from insulin insensitivity. If the muscle cells won't take them, maybe the fat cells will.

Of course they will.

Biologists say the glucose is "driven" into fat cells, which convert it, not to energy, but to glycerol, which is used to produce triglyceride. You never heard of "triglyceride"? Not by that name, perhaps, but you know it by its three-letter name, which begins with "F" and rhymes with "cat."

So when you're fit and you eat sugar, your body easily converts it into energy.

When you're not fit, your body can do nothing with it except convert it to fat for future use.

We went a little crazy when we heard about this. No wonder it's so hard for many people to lose weight—everything is stacked against them! If you're already overweight and out of shape, almost everything you eat is going to make things worse. And even when you eat less, it doesn't get much better—remember that part about your body assuming you may be starving to death, so it slows down your metabolism?

It doesn't end there.

You may think we're making the next part up, but it's all true.

When you're in good shape and you begin to exercise, the chemistry of your blood changes (it's the pH factor, for all of you who were paying attention in chemistry class.) The change in your blood chemistry actually decreases hunger *and* releases endorphins in the brain. Endorphins, you may already know, produce a natural "high." They're the body's natural painkillers. When they flood the brain, you start feeling good, your self-esteem rises and your overall attitude improves.

This is no fitness-freak's fantasy. It is a measurable scientific fact.

Once again, all of this is unfair to overweight and out-of-shape people. Their self-esteem and attitude are going nowhere but down. They become anxious and depressed. And what come naturally to anxious and depressed people? Of course: They eat. And so it goes.

This is why we want you to get aggressive about what you eat and how active you become—because the odds are stacked against you if you make only a halfhearted effort.

If it helps, go back to the page you checked off in Chapter 1 and review all those good things about yourself, and how you can make use of them. The battle's waiting to be won . . . by you.

How lifting weights affects your set point

Lifting weights doesn't burn as many extra calories as many bodybuilders may believe—you still need that aerobic activity. The benefit of weight lifting (as it affects our weight) is building muscle mass. As we saw earlier, the more muscle mass on our bodies, the more calories our bodies burn during any given activity—or inactivity. So, if you add muscle mass and maintain your intake of calories, you've already taken a major step toward reducing your set point.

And you don't need a $2,000 machine to do it either. If you can't afford a $45 set of small barbells, fill two 1-quart (1L) jugs with water or sand. And get started.

Another bonus from building muscle mass: Ever seen a muscle-bound wimp?

Remember those old Charles Atlas ads, with the cartoon of the 98-pound weakling putting up with the muscle-bound bully kicking sand in his face? They were corny but they worked—for about sixty years!

They worked, because the men (it was almost always men) who clipped the little coupon didn't necessarily want muscles galore, they just didn't want to be the kind of person who kept getting sand kicked in his face.

In other words, they wanted *attitude*. They wanted a sense of personal pride and security in what they did and what they stood for. They wanted heaps of self-esteem, and if it came with 18-inch biceps, fine.

We don't know a more self-fulfilling prophecy than attitude. In military training and business schools, candidates are always taught, "If you look like a leader, you're already a leader." That's the power of attitude, and few people accomplish anything meaningful without it.

So here's what we want you to do.

★ Lower this book, close your eyes, and visualize the person you want to become. *Don't picture someone else, like Cindy Crawford or Mel Gibson.* Picture yourself having lost weight, added muscle mass, changed your wardrobe and improved your image of yourself. Wallow in it. Wish for it. Imagine where it might lead in your career, your relationships and your life. Go ahead. Do it now. We'll be right here when you come back. (Don't forget to come back—this is just the beginning.)

★ Hello again. If you gave the image serious thought and permitted yourself to enjoy it, you're probably feeling a little excited and ready to go. But, depending on the level of your current self-esteem, you may also hear a nagging little voice saying things like: "What's the use?" "It'll take too long." And: "Who are you kidding?" We've all heard that voice before. It can make us frustrated and angry. So what happens when someone else makes you frustrated and angry? Part of you wants to yell "Shut up!" Okay, it's not very polite but at least it lets the other person know your true feelings. So, say it now, if you're hearing that voice. Say it aloud (but watch the volume level if you're reading this on the subway, or your boss is talking to someone in the background ...). Say "Shut up!" whenever that voice starts telling you "You can't succeed" or offers similar opinions. And keep saying it until the voice gets the message. Because, by that time, you will have succeeded.

★ Don't forget to reward yourself with each accomplishment. (It's best if this reward has no connection with food.) We know an overweight woman who promised herself new lingerie every time she lost 10 pounds. Nice idea. And her lingerie drawer, by the way, is overflowing.

★ Surround yourself with people who share your commitment to wellness. If this means seeing less of dedicated couch-potato friends, too bad. Now's the time to be selfish. (And when your overweight friends see the difference becoming *Armed and Dangerous* can make, they just might choose to start hanging out with you, seeking support.)

★ Put yourself first in other ways as well. If you have a favorite activity, like a brisk twenty-minute walk after dinner, don't let anyone else interfere with it. If friends or your partner need to talk to you at that time, insist they walk with you. *Be strong for yourself.*

★ Take one day at a time. You didn't become overweight and out of shape overnight; it will take a little while to turn things around. Hang on to the small improvements as measures of your success. Just hold that image in your mind—the one of you becoming the person you want to look like.

★ Control your own life. Don't give in to a change in your activity routine or a "pig-out" feast when you really don't want to. It's your life, your fat and your self-esteem you're trying to change here.

★ Hear that little voice in the background saying "You'll never do it!"? Tell it to shut up. Right now. Rotten little devil. What's it ever done for you anyway?

Check off these facts if you agree with them:

❏ I have my own definition of happiness. It's:_____

_____

❏ Physical and mental health are connected—if you improve one, you improve the other.

❏ I do not accept the idea that wanting to lose weight and look more attractive is merely a "superficial" goal.

❏ To reach the goal I want, I'll need equal quantities of low-fat eating habits, regular physical activity and a positive attitude.

❏ My body's "set point" weight is not a permanent fixture.

❏ I will not allow anyone – including me – to damage my positive attitude and self-esteem.

If you don't agree with a statement above, write your reasons here:

CHAPTER SEVEN

_____

_____

_____

_____

_____

_____

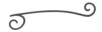

Is Male Fat Different from Female Fat?

Most books written on the topic of eating low-fat foods and staying fit are purchased by women. Which raises the question: Are women more concerned about maintaining a slim body and generally improving their health than men are?

A lot of people—almost all of them women—would answer with an enthusiastic "Darn right!" They might even offer these reasons:

★ Society values personal appearance in women more than in men—a variation on the way time treats each gender differently. ("Women get lines; men get character.")

★ Women have a more difficult time shedding excess fat than men do because women's bodies normally contain a greater ratio of fat to muscle.

★ Male activities are more prone to toning muscle than are female activities; women are social, men are competitive.

★ Fat treats women and men differently. It settles on thighs, buttocks and hips in women, and on tummies in men.

★ Some men are almost proud of their excess fat. They refer to their "beer bellies" and their "love handles" as though talking about favorite pets. They pat them lovingly and say things like "It's been a good summer!" Have you ever seen a woman gaze with pride on her too-wide hips or heavy thighs?

★ Men get hung up on everything macho. Macho means the same thing to some men that a fresh, perfect manicure means to some women. In other words, don't mess with it. Steak is macho; cottage cheese isn't. Shooting pool is macho; power-walking isn't. Beer is macho; cranberry juice isn't.

Is all of this true? Yes, for a certain kind of man—the kind who thinks women are impressed by a guy who can squeeze an empty beer can flat with his hand. Most men, we like to believe, are growing more realistic than that.

If you are married to, or just keeping company with, a man with a 1990s body and a 1950s mind and you're switching to a low-fat diet and greater activity in pursuit of wellness, congratulations. All of us, men and women alike, tend to defer somewhat to the lifestyles of our partners. We'll put our money on any woman who is determined to carve her own path toward better health.

Wife to Overweight Husband, as she watches him walk naked from the shower through the bedroom:
"Boy, you really should diet!"

Husband (looking down and trying to see beyond his large pot belly):
"Why, what color is it now?"

We've been preaching about changing things like your fat intake and activity levels for selfish reasons alone—so why is it important to be concerned about your partner's lifestyle choice? If the guy you share your life with is happiest gnawing on chicken wings and ribs every night of his life, why not let him?

We assume it's because you care enough about the big hairy butterball to want him around for a few extra years. Or maybe you're just tired of being in the presence of a man who looks like his biggest sports hero may be the Goodyear blimp.

But there are very selfish reasons as well.

We're all social beings; the actions of those we care for will influence us one way or another. If our partner shares our efforts, especially when it involves a change in lifelong habits, that's a positive influence we can use—so why not?

Still, if you're a woman and your male partner doesn't share your concerns about eating low-fat, go for it on your own. It may be difficult; it may even threaten the relationship. Trust us—last time we checked, it was easier to find another relationship than to find another life.

Macho Food = Mucho Fat

Fat Content (as a % of total calories) in meals popular among (some) North American men[1]

Braised short ribs	80 percent
Rib-eye steaks (Choice)	77 percent
Canned chili (Armour)	72 percent
Broiled T-bone steak (Choice)	68 percent
Lean spare ribs (Country-Style)	54 percent
Sausage and pepperoni pizza	51 percent
Cold beer	0 percent

Men are beginning to recognize facts that women have known for years—maybe not quickly enough, in the eyes of some women (and in the eyes of many men who don't fit the rapidly fading stereotype). But many of the wellness factors embraced by women, whether driven by health concerns or by an effort to improve

---

[1] Karen Bellerson's *The Complete and Up-To-Date Fat Book*, (Garden City Park, NY: Avery, 1993).

their appearance, are finally making an impact on men. Why? We think there are several reasons. We also believe that an intelligent male with measurable levels of testosterone and/or perception should respond to at least one of the following.

★ *Trouble at the heart of maleness.* For generations, too many men (and let's face it, many women as well) tended to ignore the connection between the foods we eat, the lives we lead and the diseases that kill us. Our modern Western lifestyle has produced higher-than-necessary death levels from heart disease, stroke and various cancers. Some of us got the message; too many of us still haven't, or got it too late.

Prostate cancer is finally catching the attention of men. Although easily cured if discovered early enough (U.S. Senator Bob Dole and super-macho military man Norman Shwarzkopf have both survived the disease), its location and function have made it difficult for men to contemplate until now, when the disease is receiving widespread attention. The prostate's position directly behind the male gonads, and its function as part of the reproduction system, both strike at the heart of a man's very identity. Most men prefer to assume they'll enjoy eternal perfection and performance from the entire region; suggesting a serious problem may exist there for years without the owner's knowledge is like speculating about a mad dog living in your basement—you can't afford to ignore it, but you'll be damned if you'll go down to check!

While some blood tests are considered effective is identifying prostate cancer, the most widely used method involves digital examination through the rectum. To women who have tolerated internal vaginal examinations and Pap smears during their adult years, this may seem merely inconvenient. To many men, it is nothing less than a torturous personal invasion, which is why early discovery of prostate cancers is so rare.

We don't really know if greater risk from prostate cancer will change the views of men who responded to warnings about lung cancer and heart disease by lighting up a cigarette. But considering that the risk involves another, more "mean-

Prostate treatment that men don't even have to bend over for:

Clinical tests have proven that eating foods low in fat reduces the incidence of prostate cancer.

But, according to a study at Memorial Sloan-Kettering Cancer Center in New York City, men may actually be able to slow the progress of prostate cancer, or even reverse the cancer growth, by switching to a diet low in fat content. Researchers were able to halt prostate tumors in laboratory mice by reducing the fat content of their diet from 40 to 21 percent or less of total calories.

Statistics already indicate that consuming minimal amounts of fat from animal sources (as found in red meats and high-fat dairy products such as cheese) can cut the chances of getting prostate cancer to 1/10th or less compared with diets high in these food groups.

ingful" part of their anatomy, it just might give them pause to think about things.

If your male partner is less than supportive about your efforts to eat food with lower levels of fat, circle the box above in red pencil and leave this book open alongside his next serving of steak and fried onions.

★ *Take the competitive route.* Men are born to be competitive in ways that women aren't. (We know: this is a generalization, and all generalizations where gender is concerned can be attacked. But, like it or not, boys and girls, it's relatively true, and we're not making a value judgment here.) Why not tap that competitive streak, if that's what it takes to get your male partner to join you in a wellness program based on low fat and higher activity? Challenge him to a goal with a reasonable (or even unreasonable) prize to the winner. You want to spend your tax return on new drapes, and he'd rather get a power saw? Fine—winner gets the choice. He wants to go skiing this winter, and you prefer Barbados? Settle it with a contest.

By the way, we don't propose saying he or she who loses the most weight wins; make it a combined target, such as weight-loss percentage and activity such as body push-ups, or entering and finishing a fun-run or charity walk. We want you both slim and fit, not anorexic. And don't forget to consult your doctor first.

★ *Go for the muscle.* Another form of competition is not from you as a woman, but from other men—imaginary or unattainable ones, of course. All right, maybe the sight of biceps the size of smoked hams isn't important to you as a woman. (We bet it is, but not as important as men think it can be.) Still, a well-muscled body has to be far more appealing than a beached-and-bleached whale—which is both an unfair but reasonably accurate description of some out-of-shape middle-aged men.

Invest in a magazine about muscle-building. Let your partner catch you reading it. Find a photo of a well-muscled male on one of the pages and hold it up, comparing his body with your partner's. Ask your partner to make a fist and bend his arm, so you can feel his biceps. If they remind you more of overripe avocados than cast-iron anvils, say nothing. Just smile sadly, sigh a little and walk away. If he asks what the problem is, tell him you still love him anyway and kiss him lightly on the cheek.

★ *Hey, we're not talking rabbit food here!* Too many people equate "low fat" with carrot sticks and tofu. Nothing wrong with them, but they don't exactly get our pulse racing either. Our foods are low-fat, not low-interest. If you or your man is wondering how you can appease your appetites on a low-fat regimen, skip ahead and scan the recipes in Chapter 10. Or just let your taste buds start fantasizing about meals that include such dishes as:

No woman ever falls in love with a man unless she has a higher opinion of him than he deserves.

L. A. STERLING

High-Brow Tarragon Chicken

A simple yet elegant dish that could form the basis
for a romantic téte-à-téte dinner.
Chill the Chardonnay!

Man-Style Chicken Loaf

Spicy honest-to-goodness meat loaf
without the high-fat content.
Toast with a cold beer!

A Better Borscht

Rich beet soup with shredded cabbage.
Soak up the rest with French bread (but hold the butter ...)!

★ ***There's always the ultimate weapon.*** We don't wish to intrude into your most intimate activities, but let's think about sex again for a moment.

Forget the fact that a tiny segment of the population are sexually aroused at the image of rolling fat on naked bodies. Some people are sexually aroused by the sight of telephone poles too. So what? We're talking normal people here.

Frankly, we think the idea of overweight men being proud of their excess fat is a lot of hooey. They may have given up the idea of losing weight and become defensive about it, or decided they would take "pride" in their obesity. That's a classic psychological response to hostility, or to feeling "different." But let's all face up to it: One way or another, our body reflects our inner feelings and values, and our inner feelings and values are expressed by our appearance—including our body shape.

There is nothing sexy about fat. It gets in the way of good sex, both figuratively and literally. It's like a feather pillow—a little of it can be comfortable but too much of it in the wrong place is

"Feeling bad about your body can affect your behavior and inhibit you both socially and sexually. . . . You seem to be always fighting the stereotyping of your body image. You may be fat, but you are not jolly. We all make assumptions according to body images. You may expect men with big noses to have big penises, and women with big breasts to be good in bed. Get to know and appreciate your body, and you can do the things for your body that you know will make you feel good."[2]

suffocating. Any way you measure sexual pleasure—by quantity, by quality, by frequency or by the kind of explosions that leave your eyes bloodshot and your toes permanently curled like fiddle-heads—it's better when you're thinner.

---

[2]Patricia E. Raley *Making Love: How to Be Your Own Sex Therapist* (New York: Dial, 1976), 81.

Check off these facts if you agree with them:

- ❏ It's important to me for my male partner to share my goals.

- ❏ I care about my male partner's good health.

- ❏ In spite of the above, I'm determined to become less fat and more fit, whether he likes it or not!

- ❏ Prostate cancer, which is linked to high-fat diets, is reason enough for my male partner to reduce his fat intake.

- ❏ Low-fat, nutritious food can still be interesting and exciting.

- ❏ Excess body fat gets in the way of a lot of things – including good sex.

If you don't agree with a statement above, write your reasons here:

_____

_____

_____

_____

_____

_____

CHAPTER EIGHT

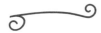

Squeezing Past the Checkout Counter

I t's almost six o'clock and you haven't thought about dinner yet. Maybe you're planning a meal just for yourself, maybe something for the two of you, maybe your whole brood is waiting for you to zap together a great meal with a flick of the refrigerator door and a quick wave of your magic food processor.

Two things you know for sure: You want to eat low-fat—no more than 25 percent of your total calorie intake from fats—and you don't want take-out food. (Frankly, we think trying to eat low-fat with take-out food is like trying to clean the wax from your ears by playing Russian roulette. . . .)

So you open the pantry and start checking things out. Pasta's good—and there's a can of marinara sauce. Might be nice over noodles . . . except canned marinara sauce is typically 45 percent fat in terms of calorie count. Hmmm. Maybe open that can of sockeye salmon, make a salad or casserole . . . Whoops—the calories in canned sockeye salmon are 50 percent fat. Okay, okay—time's a-wasting, so maybe you'll go with Hamburger Helper and there's a green bean and mushroom casserole in the freezer. Boy, that sounds healthy.

No, it sounds *fat*. The Hamburger Helper meal will hit somewhere over 40 percent fat content by calories, and the frozen casserole could score over 60 percent!

Now, before you raise this book over your head and toss it in a splendid arc toward your microwave oven in total frustration, take heart. For many people, this may be the most important and most enlightening chapter in the book. Sure, staying active is important. So is finding ways to generate a positive image of yourself, and preparing meals without fat, where possible.

But the place to start cutting back your fat intake isn't in front of your freezer or at the open door of your pantry. It's at your supermarket, as you set out down the aisle pushing that empty cart in front of you.

Hi, Wendy Here:

A few years ago, when I started consciously looking for low-fat foods, I was definitely in the minority. All around me, men and women were grabbing cans and packages off the shelves and dropping them into their carts, while I stood squinting at the backs of the labels, trying to figure the fat content.

Now I see more and more people reading the backs of labels—and, thank goodness, more and more food companies are providing nutrition information in detail. It makes it easier for all of us.

But here's what *not* to do: Please do *not* choose the food products you buy strictly on the basis of the front of the label—especially when the labels say things like "Low-Fat" or "Reduced Fat" or "Cholesterol Free." As you'll see later in this chapter, it's important to know what those phrases really mean. If the fat content of a manufacturer's standard food product is 85 percent of calories and they produce a version that's only 60 percent, they have a right to call it "Reduced Fat"—*but it's still far too high!*

"Cholesterol Free"? It probably is. Canola oil is 100 percent cholesterol-free, but it's also 100 percent oil!

So, arm yourself with the basic facts included in this chapter before setting off for the supermarket.

Sorry, but here's another legend blown all to heck.

Few foods have captured the imagination of health-conscious people more than tofu. It's high in protein (from soybean curd) and contains zero cholesterol. Very nice—except the calories in standard tofu are typically 50 percent fat! Salted and fermented versions are almost 70 percent fat! High in protein? Definitely. Health food? We don't think so. If using tofu, be sure to look for low-fat brands.

Most of us still shop the way our parents and grandparents did. We start by looking for products—canned peas, fresh milk, cold cuts, sliced bread and so on. Then we look for brand names, or, if we're bargain hunting, we look for generic or private-label products. Quantity and price are next—Will this be enough? Is the price good? When everything matches our needs, in the cart it goes.

This all happens during the few minutes it takes you to go down one aisle and up another. Behind the scenes, food manufacturers have been yanking on invisible strings attached to various parts of your anatomy, including your eyes, your heart, your taste buds and your memory for advertising messages absorbed over the days and hours before setting off on your grocery trek.

Some of those strings are purely visual—in canned goods, for example, they include label colors and photos of perfectly prepared products, hand-selected and perfectly positioned before the picture was taken. See that shade of red on the label? Teams of color researchers and marketing executives studied more shades of red than you ever knew existed before approving that particular one.

The products on the eye-level shelves are more likely to be purchased by you than those down near the floor. In fact, eye-level products are invariably the best-sellers in their category. Not only that, but some food companies actually pay the supermarkets to place their products at eye level for precisely that reason—or at the ends of aisles, where some products are likely to tumble into your cart as you round the display.

Then there are memory nudges. A string of words you may never have seen in print jumps out at you from a cereal package. The phrase suddenly comes alive as a line of music from a television commercial, and you're immediately reminded of just how good that product is reputed to taste.

Some appeals are strictly monetary, almost to the point of bribery. You like brand A of bread, but . . . Why, lookee there, Harold! Good old brand B's taking 25 cents off their loaf this week with this special coupon conveniently located right here on the shelf. So brand B it is, this week at least.

Other methods of manipulation are not quite as forthright. Over the past few years, about the only phrase that rivals a politician's election promises for lack of real meaning is the word "Light" on food-product packages—or, if you prefer, "Lite." (Why do they spell it that way? Do the food companies think that fewer letters in the word suggests fewer calories in the food? Very strange. . . .) Another good one is "Calorie Reduced!" Does this tell you all you need to know about things like fat content? Did you tell your spouse everything he or she needed to know about you on your first date?

How much lighter is "Light"?
Calorie and fat content of three U.S. national brands of butter-flavored microwave popcorn:

JOLLY TIME	195 calories	11 grams of fat
WEAVER POPCORN	195 calories	9 grams of fat
COUSIN WILLIE'S 40 percent LESS FAT		
LIGHT-RECIPE POPCORN	190 calories	8 grams of fat

Even during the shortest visit to your supermarket, you will be bombarded with messages and appeals for products and brands you probably never thought of purchasing when you entered the store. Obviously, this can have a serious effect on your grocery budget. (Which is why it's a good idea to prepare a shopping list and try—try really hard—to stick to it.) But when you're making an effort to eat low-fat and you're still acquiring the knowledge you need to choose your foods carefully, it can be disastrous. So:

Before you drop anything into your supermarket cart, study the text on the back or side of the package—the data you'll find there is much more important than the perfect photograph on the front of the label.

We mean the nutritional information. Most people who even glance at these figures rarely get past the calorie level. But remember that you'll encounter two kinds of calories: those found in sugar and carbohydrates, and those found in fat. They are two different breeds of animal, and one is definitely more dangerous than the other.

Remember, too, that it's the number of calories *from fat* that we're trying to reduce. It's wise to keep your overall caloric intake at a safe level, of course. But two slim people of similar size and activity levels can eat the same number of calories per day and, at the end of a month or so, look as different as Laurel and Hardy. (We assume, of course, that they both started out as men. . . .) The difference in weight gained will be directly related to the different source of calories in their food.

Here are two examples of nutritional information from different brands and recipes of soup. Notice that both provide 100 calories per serving. The major difference is in the fat grams.

NUTRITIONAL INFORMATION PER SERVING (270 mL)

	CAN "A"	CAN "B"
Energy	110 calories (420 kj)	110 calories (420 kj)
Protein	5 grams	6.5 grams
Fat	1 gram	8.2 grams
Polyunsaturates	0 grams	1.3 grams
Monounsaturates	0 grams	3.0 grams
Saturates	0 grams	4.0 grams
Cholesterol	0 mg	7.8 mg
Carbohydrates	22 grams	2.3 grams
Sodium	830 mg	945 mg
Potassium	200 mg	200 mg

See the "kJ" after calories? That stands for "kilojoules," another way of measuring energy. Nobody uses it instead of calories, except for a bunch of guys in a lab up north somewhere who have plastic pen protectors in their shirt pockets. Kilojoules have about as much to do with real life as Madonna's Sunday-school attendance record. We'll keep using "calories."

Both soups have 110 calories per serving—that's fairly low, and would persuade a lot of people concerned about weight reduction that these were equally good. The key thing to read here is the number of grams of fat per serving. In this case, the difference is disturbing.

Soup "A" has only 1 gram of fat; soup "B" contains 8.2 grams of fat.

Soup "A" obtains most of its calories from carbohydrates—specifically, pasta noodles. We know, because we ate the soup after reading the label. Pretty tasty, too. (Hey, it's not all fun sitting here slapping a keyboard to turn out a book, you know. . . .)

Soup "B" is a cream base, which explains the high fat content. (We ate that too—not because we necessarily enjoyed it, but because we both remembered our mothers telling us to clean our plates and to remember people in other parts of the world who would be going to bed hungry that night. Which made us suspect that maybe 65 percent of all body fat is derived from guilt.)

It's time to repeat the "9 and 4" rule to reducing fat, losing weight and following your "cruise control" setting:

> *One gram of fat contains 9 calories. One gram of carbohydrates contains 4 calories.*

So take the number of grams of fat in each brand of soup—1 gram in soup A and 8.2 grams in soup B—and multiple by 9 to measure the total number of calories from fat per serving.[1] In soup

---

[1] Not all products, of course, measure a serving size the same way. In this case, both manufacturers assumed 270 mL equals 1 serving. But some other soups may say 300 mL is a serving, or 420 mL. *The serving size doesn't count* when measuring fat from calories, because both the fat content and calorie count will rise or fall with the serving size. Don't worry about comparing serving size as long as they are reasonably close.

A, this equals 9 calories from fat; in soup B, it works out to 73.8 calories from fat (9 × 8.2). Now divide each figure by the number of calories per serving shown, and you'll arrive at this:

SOUP A 9 calories from fat divided by 110 calories = 8 percent
SOUP B 73.8 calories from fat divided by 110 calories = 67 percent

Both soups have equal numbers of calories, but one soup is two-thirds fat in its calorie count, and the other is less than 10 percent. Remember, too, that your body greets these two kinds of calories differently. When fat calories arrive in your bloodstream, the body says, "Right this way. Go directly to the hips. Do not pass Go and don't bother the liver." But when carbohydrate calories arrive, the body says, "Whoa there!" and divides them into two groups. One group is put to work right away, helping to keep your various muscles moving. The other group is sent to school, where it's graduated as fat. Then it can start its chosen career, which usually consists of destroying your self-esteem.

From soup to nuts

Sometimes cutting your fat intake is mostly a matter of changing your taste. Consider nuts as snacks, for example.

Most nuts are very high in fat content—usually 80 percent or higher.

(The winner is macadamia nuts; 1 ounce (28 g) scores 200 calories and more than 20 grams of fat, for a fat/calorie score of 95 percent!)

Ever tried roasted chestnuts? They're only 5 percent fat.

More and more food companies are providing not only the nutritional information on their labels, but also the fat content as a percentage of calories. This makes us happy and really upsets the people who make pocket calculators, because shoppers don't have to stand around punching the fat-to-calories formula (multiply grams of fat by 9 and divide by total calories) into their calculators, which makes them look like racetrack betters working out the odds-on favorite in the next race.

Still, we think it's a good idea to pack a pocket calculator in your wallet or purse when you go shopping. We also think it's a good idea to bring along our handy-dandy "Wendy and Barb's *Armed and Dangerous* Tear-Out Shopping Guide" at the end of the book. It covers the fat content of most food groups, helping you to make wise choices in your food selections.

Never trust the fat content alone.

The serving size listed by the food manufacturer on the label isn't critical. It's the percentage of calories from fat that tells you if the contents qualify for your kitchen.

As a matter of fact, we're just a trifle suspicious that some food companies use an unrealistic serving size to fool shoppers who don't do their math. Here's a good example:

We came across a new brand of tomato bruschetta, described as "The Ultimate Tomato Topper." The label also proclaimed it was "Low in Fat." Serving suggestions on the label included pouring over pasta, as a base for chicken cacciatore, and as a tomato sauce for homemade pizza. Very nice. But let's look at the nutritional information:

Energy	10.1 calories/42.2 kJ
Protein	0.2 grams
Fat	0.7 grams
Polyunsaturates	0.2 grams
Monounsaturates	0.3 grams
Saturates	0.1 grams
Cholesterol	0 mg
Carbohydrates	0.7 grams

Pretty nifty, isn't it? Just 10 calories per serving, and only 0.7 grams of fat. But look again. Multiply 0.7 grams by 9 and we have 6.3. Since each serving has just 10.1 calories, this low-fat tomato mixture is 63 percent fat!

Incidentally, the serving size is 15 grams. What's that in volume—a tablespoon? A teaspoon? A bushel and a peck? We don't know, and neither will you unless you have a good kitchen scale. But we're certain you'll pour more than 15 grams on your pizza, pasta and chicken cacciatore—which means you're pouring 63 percent fat on your food. Incidentally, the product is sold by volume in 750-mL jars, which makes it even more difficult to calculate the actual fat content per serving.

So watch yourselves. It's dangerous out there.

Notes for those who like to shop

Our whole idea in this book—and especially in this chapter—is that *we're not asking you either to starve yourself or to deprive yourself of the joy of eating most of the foods you've grown used to eating. Instead, we're asking you to make choices.*

★ First choice: Take off and keep off excess weight to make you (choose one or as many as you like) ❏ Look better; ❏ Feel better; ❏ Live better; ❏ Live longer.

★ Second choice: Support your first choice by limiting your fat intake.

★ Third choice: Understand how your body works, and why it needs less fat and more activity.

For example, almost every weight-loss diet you've ever heard about lectures against snacks. Reach for one lousy potato chip and you almost expect a big hand to come down out of the sky and slap you.

We don't buy that. We think most people can eat all the food they crave. They shouldn't push themselves away from the table wanting more to eat. And when their tummies start talking snacks, they should enjoy them.

So how do you take it off, keep it off, and become more fit? With five steps:

1. Guard with your life the 30 percent-and-under fat barrier. Don't let any of the 30+ percent fat foods into your life, let alone your mouth.

2. Discover the growing number of low-fat (under 30 percent) foods available on the market to help stifle the craving for fat.

3. When you're comfortable with the 30 percent-and-under formula, set your cruise control a little lower—at 25 percent or 20 percent.

4. Eat bulky, nutritious food that fills you up, leaves you feeling satisfied and provides your body with all the good stuff it needs to stay healthy.

5. Get yourself active—in ways that are fun and not torture.

Discover the habit of trimming the fat.

When shopping for groceries, there are other things you can do beyond following the 9-calories-per-gram-of-fat rule. In some cases, they let you enjoy foods you might think are unsuitable for a low-fat diet. Try these yourself and soon they'll become second nature:

1. *Not all pork is high in fat.* Lean pork tenderloin gets only 26 percent of its calories from fat.

2. *Not all turkey is low in fat.* Skinless turkey breast is super—less than 5 percent fat calories. But turkey bologna and turkey franks can reach up to 70 percent fat. And before you order a turkey sandwich, check to make sure it's made from pure skinless turkey breast only. So-called turkey roll can be made from different cuts of the bird with some fat added, bringing it well over the 30 percent fat level.

3. *Venison is very low in fat.* If you enjoy roast venison, eat up! Ounce for ounce, it has fewer total calories and fewer calories from fat than roasted skinless chicken breast.

4. *Trim the fat, but remember the cholesterol.* Trimming visible fat from meat and removing the skin from poultry will cut the saturated-fat content of the meat by one-half or more. Unfortunately, it does little to lower the cholesterol level of the food.

5. *Enjoy the shellfish—with caution.* If you like shrimp, eat up—four large shrimp contain a total of 0.3 grams of saturated fat. But then there's the cholesterol: 152 milligrams. (Need we say you don't dip the shrimp or lobster in melted butter? Use lemon juice or seafood sauce instead.)

6. *Great news for buttermilk lovers!* Which has less fat per serving—buttermilk or 1 percent low-fat milk? Believe it or not, it's buttermilk!

7. *Speaking of milk . . .* Popular 2 percent partially skimmed milk may be only 2 percent fat by weight, but you get 35 percent of its total calories as fat; 1 percent milk is about 23 percent fat calories.

8. *Fudge or brownie?* An ounce (28 g) of chocolate fudge has about half the fat content of a 1-ounce Brownie. (But check out our Bikini Brownies in your local store. You'll never miss the fat, and they're better than fudge.)

A supermarket shopping strategy

Believe it or not, you can start losing weight even before you leave home on your grocery-shopping trip. We've collected a list of tips to help you make healthy choices without making you feel like someone is holding a loaded gun against your head as you trundle past the deli counter. Once again, each one may seem like a small step toward losing weight and getting fit, but if the journey of a thousand miles begins with a single step (Who said that first? It was either a Chinese politician or a Royal walking out the door on his or her spouse. . . .), then the reduction of heavy thighs begins with a single gram.

And remember—this isn't a food version of self-flagellation for your sins. You want to serve a neat prime-rib roast for guests some night, go for it. Same thing for setting out a cheese tray for the bridge or poker party. Just remember to include some low-fat/no-fat items as well. By following the rules below, you'll be making important progress, step by step.

Step 1: *Prepare yourself before leaving home.* Okay, you've heard the one about making a shopping list and sticking to it. Maybe you even make a habit of never shopping for groceries immediately before a meal, knowing that an empty tummy lowers your resistance (eat a snack, like an apple or a piece of low-fat cheese if necessary).

But here are a few more hints worth remembering:

★ Give yourself plenty of time, so you can spare a few minutes to study labels before buying.

★ Bring discount coupons only for the foods you plan to buy. Otherwise, you may choose items solely on the basis of saving a few pennies instead of choosing the foods that meet your fat-content level.

★ Got kids? Leave the little angels at home when grocery shopping. They'll distract you from making the best choices and ask for high-calorie treats in voices you can't resist.

Step 2: *Favor the produce section.* Vegetables tend to demand more than their share of high-fat cooking or condiments, such as butter, sour cream and cooking oil. So set up a defense like this:

★ Choose only the freshest produce. No matter how much you may like a certain vegetable, if it ain't fresh, it ain't for you. Fresher produce not only has more nutrients, it has more flavor, which means you'll be less inclined to add a high-fat condiment.

★ Try one new fruit or vegetable every week (assuming it's fresh, of course). This way you'll widen your list of options, adding more variety and more selections when choosing freshness.

★ Salad bars in grocery stores are good time-savers, but you'll pay an extra price for the convenience. If you choose a precut salad, avoid the dressing, plus no-nos like bacon bits, croutons (most are cooked with oil) and anything that looks suspiciously like mayo.

Step 3: *Be on your guard at the dairy case.* Remember that all milk products are derived from an animal that you do not wish to be mistaken for. So take these precautions:

★ Avoid full-fat dairy products of any kind. Almost everything made with milk or cream has a low-fat alternative. Choose it whenever possible.

★ If you or your family simply cannot stomach skim milk, look for brands that use a special filtering system to reduce the time spent in pasteurization. It really does improve the flavor—2 percent tastes like homogenized, 1 percent tastes like 2 percent and skim tastes terrific! (In Canada, these brands are Neilson's and Lactantia Pure Filter.)

★ Run, run, run away from "non-dairy" creamers. They're no lower in fat than regular dairy products and they often replace the cream with coconut or palm oils, which will boot your cholesterol level upstairs.

★ Low-fat yogurts are fine, but some of the fruit-flavored ones have a high sugar content. Suggestion: Choose plain yogurt and add your own fresh fruit.

★ Some cheeses call themselves "Partly skimmed." That's a little like calling yourself partly pregnant—it may not show right now, but later the truth will be obvious. Even partly skimmed cheeses can contain fat levels of 60 percent or more.

Step 4: *Stay in the light near the meat counter.* We think eating much less red meat is a good idea for everyone, and you'll get no argument about that from the cows either. But whatever meats you choose, use these rules as a guide:

★ Buy meat only when you have a special recipe in mind. If you're looking for a recipe using red meat, make it one that cooks the meat in the presence of moisture. Then you can choose cuts with a lower fat content, such as round steak or loins.

★ When buying pork, lamb or veal, the cuts labeled "loin" and "leg" are lower in fat.

★ Your best choice at the poultry counter is skinless white meat. We know, it's also the most expensive. Life is unfair. You can always remove the skin yourself, either before or after cooking. If that saves you money, go for it.

★ Self-basting poultry? Sure—after the bird bastes itself, it bastes you from the inside. These things are loaded with added fat—keep walking.

★ Cold cuts, hot dogs and sausages may be made with chicken or turkey, but that doesn't mean they're signifi-cantly lower in fat. Always check the label.

★ Ground poultry is a fine choice for burgers, but beware if it appears too dark in color—it may mean that the butcher has included skin and dark meat, which raises the fat content. Try to buy ground white meat only.

Step 5: *Don't let fish tip the scales on you.* We should all eat more fish, as long as we choose it carefully and prepare it correctly.

★ Generally, any fish with white flesh is low in fat.

★ All shellfish is low in fat (but high in cholesterol). Just don't deep-fry them, and serve only with lemon juice or seafood sauce. Forget butter and tartar sauces.

★ Processed fish sticks, crab cakes and similar dishes are usually high in added fat, so beware.

Step 6: *Remain cool near the freezer section.* Frankly, we prefer fresh. But when convenience is number one on your list, frozen foods often can't be avoided.

★ Check the labels for your fat-content "cruise control" setting; reject anything above 30 percent fat from calories.

★ Buy only naked frozen vegetables; you can dress them up at home later with lemon juice and spices.

★ Watch out for tofu-based and non-dairy frozen desserts, unless their stated fat content is sufficiently low. (They tend to be very high in fat from other sources.)

Step 7: *Stroll up and down the aisles keeping a watchful eye.*

★ The best buys in the entire supermarket, based on price and nutrition, are dried beans, lentils, split peas and so on. High in protein and fiber, they're also fat-free.

★ We love bakeries, and you probably do as well. But as a rule, try to choose only whole-grain breads, bagels and English muffins. Corn breads, biscuits, bran muffins and refrigerated dough tend to have high fat levels, so check their labels carefully.

★ Most pastries still contain high levels of fat, although a few companies are searching for alternatives. (We're one of them; our Double Chocolate Mint Meltaway Cookies and muffins are less than 30 percent fat—about half the normal levels.) If you can't locate low-fat muffins and cookies but still want a snack with your coffee, look for fig bars, raisin biscuits and graham crackers.

★ Fat-free snacks include baked (not deep-fried) potato chips and tortilla chips, melba toast, pretzels, rice cakes and matzo crackers.

★ You can dress up fat-free snacks with all sorts of fat-free condiments such as hummus, baba-ghanouj, bruschetta, ketchup, flavored mustards (use sparingly—most are 50 percent or more calories from fat), Worcestershire sauce, soy sauce, hot sauces, butter-flavored granules and salsa. We love 'em all. Just be sure to check the sodium content if you have a problem with that ingredient.

Learning a second language— we're talking food labels here.

Sometimes you almost get the feeling that English is a second language to the people who package foods, especially when it comes to measuring fat content. What's the difference between "Low," "Lean" and "Light/Lite" anyway?

We were surprised—and delighted—to discover there really is a method to all this label madness, as defined by the U.S. Food and Drug Administration. So in case you wondered if there really were definitions for these terms, here they are:

★ *FREE, as in "Fat-free," "Calorie-free," "Sodium-free," etc.* One serving contains such a low amount of whatever goes with "free" that it doesn't mean much. "Fat-free" means less than 0.5 grams of fat per serving.

★ *GOOD SOURCE, as in "Good source of vitamin C."* One serving contains from 10 percent to 19 percent of the recom-mended daily intake of that particular nutrient.

★ *HIGH IN, as in "High in calcium."* One serving contains 20 percent or more of whatever follows "High in."

★ **LEAN and EXTRA LEAN.** Now we're talking fat content. This is used only with meats, seafood, poultry and game and tells you the following:

"Lean" contains fewer than 10 grams of total fat, fewer than 4 grams of saturated fat and fewer than 95 milligrams of cholesterol per serving.

"Extra Lean" contains fewer than 5 grams of total fat, fewer than 2 grams of saturated fat and fewer than 95 milligrams of cholesterol per serving.

★ **LIGHT and LITE.** Be careful with these guys. When used on their own, they indicate that one serving contains one-third fewer calories and/or half the fat normally found in this product. It also indicates that sodium content has been cut by half as well. But when coupled with the product name itself—as in *"Lite Olive Oil"*—it indicates only a change in color or texture. The fat content (in the case of oil) remains at 100 percent.

★ **LOW, as in "Low fat," "Low cholesterol," etc.** This word tells you the product has reduced levels of a specific ingredient or quality. But other factors could remain high. For example, a "Low fat" product could still be high in calories, and a "Low calorie" product high in fat. Still, the manufacturers cannot use this term unless they qualify as follows (all levels are per serving):

"Low calorie" means 40 calories or less.

"Low fat" means 3 grams or less of total fat.

"Low saturated fat" means 1 gram or less of saturated fat.

"Low cholesterol" means less than 20 milligrams of cholesterol.

"Low sodium" means less than 140 milligrams of sodium.

"Very low sodium" means less than 35 milligrams of sodium.

★ **MORE, as in "More iron."** A serving portion contains 10 percent or more of the recommended daily intake of the nutrient than the brand's regular product.

★ **(PERCENT) FAT-FREE.** This designation can be used only on products already labeled as "Low-fat" or "Fat-free" and is a trifle confusing. If a 100-gram serving contains 5 grams of fat, it can be labeled "95 percent fat-free". Aha—but if the serving has 90 calories in total, that means 50 percent of its energy is derived from fat (5 times 9=45 divided by 90). So 95 percent fat-free can still be too high for your low-fat meal.

★ **REDUCED or LESS, as in "reduced fat."** Watch yourself with this one. The guidelines say anything that claims to be "reduced" or "less" must contain at least 25 percent less of that nutrient or ingredient than found in a "reference food." What's a reference food? No, it's not something you eat in a library. It can be either the company's regular product or an entirely different product that the food is being compared with. For example: "Our potato chips have 25 percent less fat!" Less than what? And less than whose? And where does that leave the fat content?

We don't mean to be harsh on food companies. (Hey, we're in the food business ourselves!) There are many rules about producing and selling food products, all designed to protect consumers. But when it comes to labels, the companies are interested primarily in reaching out a long graphic arm from the shelves to grab your sleeve and pull you toward them.

Just remember what your mother said about sweet-talking strangers.

Choose your battles carefully.

We titled our book *Armed and Dangerous* because most of us are waging war against fat. We have to fight that ugly stuff every step of the way, which can be difficult because it has a lot of allies. From food companies to our own taste buds, fat has many friends in high places.

You can choose one of two ways to win the battle against fat when it comes to shopping, cooking and choosing your foods.

One approach is total war. This means you're prepared to blast away at excess fat wherever you find it, and convince your own taste buds that fat is poison. This works very well for dedicated athletes, former monks and people who worship stones in the desert.

The other approach is to choose your battles carefully. In other words, give in to one or two *small* weaknesses and exchange those losses for strength in other places.

CHAPTER NINE

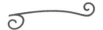

Does It Have to Contain Fat to Taste Good?

In 1995, we read a newspaper story of a series of medical seminars taking place in the southern United States. Most of the participants were young doctors learning aspects of wellness they could pass on to their patients after a week of listening, taking notes and discussing the topic.

One of the seminars attended by the reporter covering the event focused on the dangers of excess fat in American diets. Charts were flashed on the screen showing the increased risk of major diseases attributed to high levels of fat in the body. Detailed analyses of the effects of fat on physical wellness were documented. Major father-figures and mother-figures of U.S. medicine shook their fingers at the audience in warning about high fat. The reporter took notes and moved on.

During the afternoon's free session, when those attending the seminars could do whatever they wished, the reporter happened to pass a popular hamburger chain and glance inside.

She was flabbergasted.

Four participants from the session on fat dangers were grouped in a booth, attacking cheeseburgers and french fries with wild abandon. The reporter entered, introduced herself, and asked how these young medical people could do such a thing on the same day they had attended a lecture on the dangers of high-fat content in our foods.

Maybe the reporter expected a response about experimentation. Or a lost bet. Or even a little embarrassment at being caught performing a moderately indecent act.

She got none of the above. Instead, all four doctors laughed, shrugged and replied with variations on the same line: "It just tastes good!" Well. The reporter was scandalized. But we weren't. Hey, the young doctors were just proving they're as human as the rest of us.

"It just tastes good!"

What they meant was that just because something is sinful doesn't mean it's painful. In fact, aren't most sins fun in one way or another? Heck, if sins *weren't* fun, we'd all be saints!

But it started us thinking: Why do we crave so much fat in our foods? Why do we all have trouble overcoming the urge to eat foods that are high in fat content when we know they're so bad for us? Is fat addictive, like nicotine and heroin? So we did some research. We tore through all the books and magazine articles we could find on the subject. We talked to nutritionists. We talked to people who attend our seminars. And we talked to ourselves. Finally, we arrived at a bunch of conclusions:

★ ***It's an evolutionary hangover.*** Supermarkets were scarce a few eons ago. When our ancestors were living in caves and wearing bear skins, a balanced diet probably meant not being eaten by something you were trying to eat yourself. You could gorge on nuts, seeds and fruit perhaps four months out of twelve. After that, it was barbecued squirrel or nothing. So anyone whose body had both an urge and an ability to absorb quantities of fat had a better chance of surviving normal risks such as drought, winter and attacks from saber-toothed tigers. Some of those same genes remain in our bodies long after they're needed.

★ ***It's an acquired habit.*** Fat may or may not be addictive, depending on your medical training, your current weight and the number of crash diets you've attempted.

But it can certainly become a habit. Enjoying bacon and eggs in the morning and roast beef for Sunday dinner is still a pleasant memory for many middle-aged people. Never mind the risks and dangers—it was comfort food, prepared by our mothers, and some of us still miss it.

★ *We're a fast-food culture.* From take-out foods to drive-in restaurants to frozen entrées, fast foods are the norm instead of the exception for many people today. Given the pace and demands of modern life, we can't expect to change things (but it's interesting that some enlightened fast-food outlets are beginning to respond with low-fat selections). Fat continues to be a major component of convenience foods for a lot of reasons, including speed (frying is faster than baking), cost (griddles are cheaper than ovens), and—

★ *It just tastes good!* Okay, but why? Habit and genetics are two reasons; we've found a third. Fats and oils perform a key function in cooking. They actually carry the flavor of the food to our mouths. There they add texture as well. Many foods prepared without a minimum level of fat can seem dry and unappetizing to us.

We can't change genetics. But we can avoid fast foods unless they measure up (or down) to our "cruise control" setting, and we can break the habit of incorporating large quantities of fat in our diet.

It all begins, as we said earlier, in the supermarket, when we select our foods, and in our kitchen, when we prepare them.

The next chapter includes several dozen knock-out recipes that are so tasty you'll never miss the fat. But you may already have your own favorite recipes. Do you have to give them up to reduce the fat content of your diet? Not necessarily.

Below are some tips worth clipping and saving. Tuck them into your favorite cookbook—the one you won't toss out, now that you have your own copy of *Armed and Dangerous*—and make use of them. They'll help you break the high-fat habit.

SOME FOODS LIKE IT HOT

When using low-fat vinaigrette on pasta, rice, potatoes or beans, add it while the food is still warm, even if you're serving it cold. It intensifies the flavor, disguising the absence (or low level) of fat.

HIDE THE EVIDENCE

By increasing the amount of spices and condiments in your recipes, you can disguise the lowered fat content. Use larger measures of spices, herbs, vinegars and mustards, and experiment with garlic, ginger, lime, lemon, chilies and other strong flavors.

RICHER MILK WITHOUT MORE MILK FAT

When a recipe calls for whole milk, use skim milk instead. Swirl a tablespoon or so of non-fat powdered milk into each cup of skim milk for more body.

TRY UNUSUAL NON-FAT SUBSTITUTES

In your next recipe that calls for butter or margarine, try replacing all that fat with pureed prunes or other preserves. Really! Pick up a jar in the Baby Food section. They'll add the texture you want from butter in the recipe while eliminating all the fat . . . and adding a little roughage to your diet.

KNOW WHERE TO BAN FAT AND WHEN

Some measures of fat are needed in cooking. For example, the cellulose in onions and scallions starts breaking down, releasing all the flavors, only when sautéed in fat. Use a minimum of oil when required.

EGGS ARE FINE, BUT YOLKS AREN'T FUNNY

One of the easiest ways to cut the fat content in a recipe calling for whole eggs is to use more egg whites. If a recipe calls for 4 eggs, use 2 whole eggs plus 3 or 4 egg whites, and cut the fat content from eggs by 50 percent.

REMOVE THE CHICKEN SKIN AFTER COOKING

Unless a recipe calls for skinless chicken, leave the skin on for cooking. First, remove all visible fat, then cook with the skin on and remove the skin before serving. This works especially for roasting, grilling and sautéing.

CREAMY SOUPS WITHOUT CREAM #1

One chef we know makes Clam Chowder without cream. He boils quartered potatoes separately and purees half of them in a blender, adding the other half to the chowder whole. The puree makes the soup rich and creamy. You can try this with other creamed soups as well.

CREAMY SOUPS WITHOUT CREAM #2

Start actively looking for ways to cut fat and replace the flavor with other suitable ingredients. Example: If a recipe calls for a cup of heavy cream, try replacing half or more of the cream with chicken or vegetable stock instead.

CARROTS KEEP IT LEAN AND MEAN.

If you simply must use ground beef in meatballs (we think lean ground turkey is a better choice), be sure to choose extra-lean beef. Then add moisture with raw grated potato or carrot.

NEVER SUBSTITUTE A CROISSANT FOR BREAD

Most bread is low in fat—about 1 gram per slice. But avoid making sandwiches from croissants, which (since butter is a major ingredient) can score a whopping 14 grams of fat.

ATTENTION CHOCOHOLICS.

Baking chocolate is exceptionally high in fat (unsweetened chocolate for baking can reach 96 percent!). Try substituting cocoa powder instead. Three tablespoons (45 mL) of cocoa powder equal one square of baking chocolate.

INVEST IN A NON-STICK FRY PAN

If you don't already own one, purchase a non-stick pan today. If you need to be "weaned" to non-fat cooking, dampen a paper towel with Canola oil and wipe the surface before heating. This way you'll use an absolute minimum amount of oil.

Sometimes where and how you eat is as important as what you eat.

We're all creatures of habit, especially when it comes to eating. In fact, breaking our habit of eating in certain places and at certain times may be as difficult as changing the foods we put on our plates.

For example, in our harried lives, a lot of us eat while seated in front of the television, catching up on the day's disasters—also known as "the news." Trouble is, we're not concentrating on our food, which means we may tend to eat more of the wrong things.

We all know that negative emotions can lead to overeating, or eating excessive amounts of the wrong foods. So, doesn't it make sense that creating positive feelings will work the other way? Depressing surroundings—a kitchen overloaded with dirty dishes and the remains of dinner in pots on the stove, for example—are an invitation to overindulge. Try making your meals as attractive to your eyes and ears as they are to your tummy and see if you don't enjoy your food more while eating less fat.

Schedule Your Activity to Reduce Your Appetite
We'll deal with this in greater detail later, but if you exercise or plan some physical activity late in the afternoon, this can actually reduce your appetite at dinner time.

Here's another hint: After you've served your meal and before you start eating, *put the leftovers in the refrigerator while they're still warm!* We know, you've probably been told not to do that because it puts an extra load on the fridge motor or some such thing. Hogwash. If your refrigerator can't cool down a bowl of mashed potatoes and some grilled chicken without blowing a gasket, it's in far worse shape than you'll ever be! The idea, of course, is that you won't be so tempted to *schlep* out to the kitchen for a second helping if the food's already cold.

Does getting out of your kitchen mean stepping off the low-fat express?

It's hard enough controlling your fat intake when preparing meals at home. But what happens when you put yourself in the hands of somebody else who's doing the cooking?

We've already suggested calling ahead when making restaurant reservations to inquire about low-fat or no-fat entrées. But if you pop into a restaurant without reservations and no knowledge of their menu, what happens to your battle strategy?

If the restaurant cannot or will not cooperate in helping you lower your fat, relax. Being a pioneer is always a challenge. So it's time to take some defensive action. Look over the menu carefully and try to follow these rules:

★ If you expect to be dining out at a restaurant with limited low-fat choices, eat a no-fat snack before leaving the house. A banana or cup of no-fat yogurt is a good defense against being ambushed by a high-fat menu.

★ Choose grilled lean meats, chicken or fish. Grilled fish is excellent, but avoid Atlantic salmon and orange roughy—they're very high in fat (40 percent and 50 percent, respectively). Swordfish is borderline (30 percent of its calories are from fat). Some good choices—grilled, baked or broiled, of course—are light tuna, halibut and cod.

★ Insist on vegetables prepared without butter.

★ Baked potato is fine. If you find it dry, ask for yogurt and herbs instead of butter or sour cream.

★ Insist on having all salad dressings (if they're not the no-fat variety) and sauces served separately. Then apply them sparingly.

★ Avoid garlic bread, which tends to contain maximum amounts of both garlic and butter.

★ Avoid buffets—they're the terrorist sectors in low-fat/lose-weight societies, out to destroy all your plans with too much food, about which you know too little.

★ Always order half-portions, if available.

★ Pasta by itself is not fattening, but remember to ask for the sauce to be served separately. Start by adding a minimal amount, then a little more as needed. The idea is to *stay in control of the foods you ingest.*

★ Substitute tomato sauces for cream sauces on pasta.

Use TV to open your eyes.

If you still wonder why it's so difficult to lose weight, do this: Watch for food commercials—fast food (fried chicken, hamburgers, deep-fried fish, double-cheese pizza) and foods for your kitchen (salad dressings, frozen entrées, sauce for "thick juicy" steaks, etc.). Each time you see a food commercial, assess the fat content in your mind. In almost every case, the calories from fat will be 50 percent or more. With promotion like that, it's no surprise that so many of us have difficulty losing weight. . . .

Know your enemy—it's not the food groups but the food types to watch.

One of the most confusing parts about choosing low-fat foods is assuming that *all* types of a certain food are taboo in a low-fat diet. It's not really true. Not all cheese is high in fat, and not all yogurt is low in fat.

It may take a while to spot the danger areas in certain foods, but it's reassuring to know you may not have to alter your meals as much as you might have expected.

We've put together some figures on fat content in common food groups as a guide. We've also indicated saturated-fat levels—the ones to avoid for overall improved health.

1. *Beef.* This is a real danger zone. The best solution is to avoid red meat altogether, which may be tough to do for some people. Next best: Eat it as a special treat and choose low-fat cuts. Here are the fat contents for cooked beef, assuming 4-ounce (112-gram) portions:

FAT CONTENTS OF COOKED BEEF

	Calories	Fat (g)	Saturated Fat (g)
All-beef hot dog	360	32	14
Brisket, trimmed	275	14	7
Chuck roast	443	35	15
Corned beef	287	22	7
Ground beef, lean	306	20	8
Ground beef, regular	333	21	9
Pastrami	399	33	12
Prime rib	320	22	9
Rib eye	337	24	10
Salami	299	24	10
Sirloin	238	10	4
T-bone	245	12	5
Tenderloin	240	13	4
Top loin	387	29	12

2. *Poultry.* When it comes to eating low-fat meat, turkey is a real buddy. Note the difference between dark meat and light meat though, and the high fat content of poultry skin. Geese and ducks are to be avoided. Besides, we like ducks when they're alive—they're such neat, friendly creatures. We're talking 4-ounce (112-gram) portions of roasted bird here:

FAT CONTENTS OF COOKED POULTRY

	Calories	Fat (g)	Saturated Fat (g)
Chicken			
Dark meat with skin	239	18	5
Dark meat, no skin	234	11	3
Light meat with skin	254	12	3
Light meat, no skin	198	5	1
Turkey			
Dark meat with skin	253	13	4
Dark meat, no skin	214	8	3
Light meat with skin	225	9	3
Light meat, no skin	179	4	1
Goose			
With skin	349	25	8
Duck			
With skin	385	32	11

3. *Fish.* Most are low-fat, until you drizzle them with butter or Hollandaise sauce. True fish fans stick to lemon juice to bring out the full flavor. And beware of some high-fat fish masquerading as low-fat good guys. Again, we're talking 4-ounce (112-gram) portions, baked or broiled.

FAT CONTENTS OF COOKED FISH

	Calories	Fat (g)	Saturated Fat (g)
Clams	169	2	0
Cod	120	1	0
Crab, Alaskan King	111	2	0
Haddock	128	1	0
Halibut	160	3	0

	Calories	Fat (g)	Saturated Fat (g)
Lobster	112	1	0
Mackerel	299	21	5
Oysters	157	6	1
Perch	134	1	0
Pike	129	1	0
Salmon			
Pink, canned	159	7	2
Atlantic	230	8	2
Sardines in oil	238	13	3
Scallops	128	1	0
Snapper	146	2	0
Squid	200	8	2
Swordfish	177	6	2
Trout	173	5	1
Tuna			
Light, canned in oil	226	9	2
Light, canned in water	150	2	0
Light, steak	210	7	0

4. *Milk.* There's probably no more confusing food measurement than the fat content of milk. Think of 2 percent homogenized milk. Sounds good, doesn't it? Only 2 percent butterfat. Except that it equals 38 percent calories from fat, well above the 30 percent maximum for most people. Below are calorie and fat ratings for an 8-ounce (250-mL) glass.

5. *Cheese.* We love cheese! And we won't give it up completely. You don't have to either, as long as you view it as a special treat and not an eat-every-day staple on your table. Of course, choose low-fat cottage cheese. As for the others, keep reminding yourself that most cheeses score 60 to 80 percent in fat calories, and that's just too high. These are 1-ounce (28-gram) portions, except where noted:

FAT CONTENTS OF MILK

	Calories	Fat (g)	Fat%	Sat. Fat (g)
Whole milk (3% fat)	150	8	48	5
Low-fat (2%)	120	5	38	4
Low-fat (1%)	100	3	27	2
Skim	80	Trace	5	Trace
Buttermilk (1%)	100	2	18	1
Dry	80	Trace	5	Trace
Evaporated	340	20	53	17
Lactaid (1%)	100	2	18	2
Goat's milk (whole)	168	10	54	6

FAT CONTENTS OF CHEESE

	Calories	Fat (g)	Fat%	Sat. Fat (g)
Blue	100	8	72	5
Camembert/Brie	85	7	74	5
Cheddar	115	9	70	6
Cottage (1/2 cup)				
Creamed	108	5	43	3
Low-fat	104	2	17	1
Cream	100	10	90	6
Feta	75	6	72	4
Mozzarella				
Whole milk	80	6	68	4
Partly skimmed	80	5	56	3
Neufchatel	74	7	85	4
Parmesan	130	9	62	5
Ricotta				
Whole milk	216	16	66	10
Partly skimmed	170	10	53	6
Swiss	105	8	67	5

6. Yogurt. Prepared yogurt tends to be naturally low in calories, but it varies widely from brand to brand. Here are some examples. Beyond fat content, we also find that yogurt varies widely in taste and texture as well; some low-fat yogurts taste richer than their high-fat cousins. Anyway, here are a few popular yogurt brands and types selected from Karen Bellerson's *The Complete and Up-to-Date Fat Book*.[1]

FAT CONTENTS OF YOGURT

	Amount (oz.)	Fat (g)	Calories%	Fat%
Bon Lait	6	5	200	23
Dannon Fruit-on-the-Bottom				
Low-Fat Banana	8	3	240	11
Low-Fat Coffee	8	3	200	14
Low-Fat Plain	8	4	140	26
Dannon Light	8	0	100	0
Del Monte Awesome (Peach)	4.75	2	140	13
Light N'Lively				
Free (Blueberry)	4.4	0	50	0
99% Fat Free (Peach)	5	2	150	12
100 no sugar (Peach)	8	0	100	0
Original (Peach)	8	2	240	8
Yoplait				
Custard Style (Banana)	6	4	190	19
Light/Non-fat (Peach)	6	0	80	0
Low-Fat (Blueberry)	6	4	230	16
Low-Fat Breakfast	6	3	220	12
New Light/Non-Fat	4	0	60	0
Non-Fat (Plain)	8	0	120	0
Original (Peach)	6	4	190	19

[1](Garden City Park, NY: Avery, 1993).

CHAPTER TEN

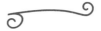

Meals to Live For

Here's where we put our money where our mouths are—literally. It's fine to identify low-fat food items on their own, but how do you put them together in nutritious recipes that never have a hint of denial?

We've assembled some outstanding recipes from friends, family and strangers who've attended our seminars and wanted to share their low-fat meal ideas with us. We tried to combine simplicity with elegance, and may even surprise you with dishes you never expected to prepare as part of a low-fat menu.

Fat content varies, and we identify the fat calories at the end of every recipe. In every case, the number of calories derived from fat is lower than 30 percent.

BREAKFAST

Spicy Baked Omelet

Another omelet favorite. The spices and salsa give this dish a sophisticated boost that makes traditional bacon and eggs sound barbaric—and maybe they are! Make a large batch of "My Sister's Salsa" (page 169). Or serve with a tossed salad and fat-free dressing, fresh French bread and cold Chardonnay, and you've got an elegant brunch or a classy summer's-day dinner. Serves 6.

1	medium onion, chopped	1
½ cup	Alpine Lace Lo mozzarella cheese	125 mL
1½ cups	skim milk	375 mL
2	whole eggs plus 3 egg whites	2
⅓ cup	all-purpose flour	80 mL
½ teaspoon	baking powder	2.5 mL
½ teaspoon	basil	2.5 mL
½ teaspoon	oregano	2.5 mL
¼ teaspoon	salt	1.25 mL
	dash Louisiana Hot Sauce	
¾ cup	"My Sister's Salsa"	180 mL

Preheat oven to 350° F (175°C). Spray 9-inch (22.5-cm) pie plate with non-stick spray. Sprinkle onion and cheese on bottom of plate.

Place remaining ingredients except salsa in a blender; cover and puree at medium-high speed for 30 seconds, or until smooth. Pour into pie plate.

Bake about 40 minutes, or until a knife inserted in omelet comes out clean. Let stand 5 minutes, then cut into wedges. Serve with a spoonful of salsa on top of each wedge.

Per serving: *Calories:* 100   *Total fat:* 2 grams
% calories from fat: 18   *Carbohydrates:* 13 grams   *Protein:* 9 grams

Muskoka-Style French Toast

Some people have a foolish way of not minding, or pretending not to mind, what they eat. For my part, I mind my belly very studiously, and very carefully; for I look upon it, that he who does not mind his belly will hardly mind anything else.

DR. SAMUEL
JOHNSON, 1763

What's this? French Toast in a low-fat cook book? Sure—the secret's in baking, not frying the toast. An extra benefit: You can squeeze all 12 slices on one cookie sheet and make a family-sized batch all at once. If you prefer, substitute ¾ cup (180 mL) Egg Beaters for the egg whites. Serves 4.

6	egg whites	6
12	slices whole wheat bread, sliced 1 inch (2.5 cm) thick	12
2 cups	cornflakes (frosted or plain)	500 mL

Beat eggs until foamy. Crush cornflakes slightly. Dip bread in egg mixture and cornflakes. Place on baking sheet. Broil until golden brown on each side. Top with sliced bananas, strawberries or maple syrup.

Per serving (1 slice): *Calories:* 200   *Total fat:* 1.2 grams
% calories from fat: 0.5   *Carbohydrates:* 55 grams   *Protein:* 8 grams

"I Can't Believe They're Legal!" Cinnamon Rolls

Sometimes even we admit that a little margarine can go a long way in improving things. In this case, 1 tablespoon (15 mL) of margarine (use the soft Canola-based variety) is divided among 8 rolls—not bad. Watch the calories though—at 300 per roll, one of these plus juice and coffee is all you need. Makes 8 rolls.

1 tablespoon	margarine	15 mL
3½ cups	all-purpose flour	875 mL
1 tablespoon	baking powder	15 mL
½ teaspoon	salt	2.5 mL
1 cup	buttermilk	250 mL
3	egg whites	3 mL
1 cup	seedless golden raisins	250 mL
¾ cup	unsweetened applesauce	180 mL
1 tablespoon	brown sugar	15 mL
2 teaspoons	cinnamon	10 mL
2 tablespoons	strawberry spreadable fruit (or "Doublefruit" jam)	30 mL

Preheat oven to 400°F (230°C). Spray baking pan 13 × 9 × 2 inches (32.5 × 22.5 × 5.0 cm) deep with non-stick coating.

Cut margarine into flour, baking powder and salt in large bowl (criss-crossing mixture with two knives). Mix in buttermilk and egg whites.

Turn dough onto floured surface and knead gently until dough is soft and easy to handle. Roll dough into a 10-inch (25-cm) square.

Mix raisins, applesauce, brown sugar and cinnamon. Spread over top of dough, then roll up dough, pinching the edge to seal mixture.

Cut into 8 slices, place in pan with the cut side up and bake 20 to 25 minutes, or until light brown. Brush tops with jam, remove from pan, and cool on wire rack.

Per serving (1 roll): *Calories:* 300 *Total fat:* 3 grams
% calories from fat: 9 *Carbohydrates:* 65 grams *Protein:* 9 grams

Judy's Coffee-Break Carrot Muffins

We got this recipe from our friend Judy Reynolds, who says they're perfect for breakfast with juice and coffee, or as a late-night snack with a glass of skim milk. The prune puree may be refrigerated up to 2 months. Makes 18 muffins.

	Non-stick cooking spray	
4 cups	peeled grated carrots	1 L
1 cup	granulated sugar	250 mL
1 cup	packed brown sugar	250 mL
1	can (8 ounces/250 mL) crushed pineapple in unsweetened juice	1
1 cup	prune puree	250 mL
4	egg whites	4
2 teaspoons	vanilla	10 mL
2 cups	all-purpose flour	500 mL
2 teaspoons	baking soda	10 mL
2 teaspoons	cinnamon	10 mL
$1/2$ teaspoon	salt	2.5 mL
$3/4$ cup	raisins	175 mL

Prune Puree (makes 2 cups)

$2^2/_3$ cup	(16 ounces/500 mL) pitted prunes	
$3/4$ cup	water	175 mL

Process 1 minute in food processor until pureed

Preheat oven to 375°F (190°C). Spray 2¾-inch muffin pan cups with non-stick spray. In bowl, combine carrots, sugar, pineapple, prune puree, eggs and vanilla. Blend thoroughly; add remaining ingredients except raisins. Mix just to blend. Add raisins. Spoon into muffin cups equally. Bake 20 minutes or until toothpick inserted in center comes out clean.

Per serving (1 muffin):   *Calories:* 187   *Total fat:* 0 grams
% calories from fat: 0   *Carbohydrates:* 45 grams   *Protein:* 3 grams

Apple-Raisin Flan

This freezes beautifully! Make some in the fall, when apples are plentiful (try to use Spys or MacIntoshes), freeze, and microwave on a cold winter's morning. Serve warm with a scoop of fat-free yogurt and some steaming black coffee. Serves 6.

3	large apples	3
¼ cup	raisins	60 mL
2 tablespoons	lemon juice	30 mL
1 teaspoon	cinnamon	5 mL
1½ cups	skim milk	375 mL
2	egg whites	2
1	whole egg	1
¼ cup	sugar	60 mL
1 teaspoon	vanilla	5 mL

Preheat oven to 350°F (175°C). Peel, core and slice apples. Toss with raisins, lemon juice and cinnamon in a large bowl.

Combine remaining ingredients separately.

Pour apple/raisin mixture into a non-stick pie plate (or use non-stick spray) and cover with milk mixture.

Bake for 50 minutes or until custard is set. Cool 15 minutes before serving.

Per serving: *Calories:* 150   *Total fat:* 1.1 grams
% calories from fat: 7   *Carbohydrates:* 13.1 grams
Protein: 4.4 grams

Appetizers 'n Tempters

Spicy Tuna 'n Bean Dip

Serve this with low-fat crackers or pita-bread squares. By the way, it also makes a great sandwich in fresh pita. You can eliminate the olive oil if you like, but, with only 17 percent fat calories, this is still a delicious low-fat party snack and appetizer. Save time and mix in a blender—you'll also get a smoother texture. Makes about 2 cups (500 mL); allow ¼ cup (60 mL) per serving.

1	6½ oz (182 g) can water-packed tuna	1
1 cup	canned white kidney beans (cannellini)	250 mL
1	stalk celery, finely chopped	1
⅓ cup	chopped onion (Spanish or red)	80 mL
1 tablespoon	lemon juice	15 mL
1 tablespoon	Dijon mustard	15 mL
1 teaspoon	olive oil	5 mL
½ teaspoon	celery seed	2.5 mL
	Dash hot pepper sauce	

Rinse and drain tuna and kidney beans. Blend lightly (or mash in a bowl with a fork). Add remaining ingredients and blend until smooth.

Per serving: *Calories:* 73   *Total fat:* 1.4 grams
% calories from fat: 17   *Carbohydrates:* 6.7 grams   *Protein:* 8.3 grams

Nicki's Saucy Meatballs

Hi, it's Barb. My sister-in-law serves these at every party she throws, and they're always a hit. The women at the party take a look at Nicki's hour-glass figure and assume that she never eats these things— but she does! (Hey, maybe if we eat more of them, we'll all have figures like Nicki's.) Serves 4.

Meatballs

2 pounds	ground turkey	900 g
1 tablespoon	flour	15 mL
1 tablespoon	milk	15 mL
	Salt and pepper to taste	

Sauce

1	12 oz (375 mL) jar Heinz chili sauce	1
1/2	6 oz (180 mL) jar grape jelly	1/2
1 teaspoon	ground cinnamon	5 mL

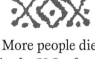

More people die in the U.S. of too much food than of too little.

JOHN KENNETH GALBRAITH, *THE AFFLUENT SOCIETY* (1957)

Preheat oven to 350°F (175°C). Mix turkey, flour, milk salt and pepper together well. Shape into cocktail-sized meat balls. Arrange on a baking sheet and bake 20–25 minutes, or until evenly brown.

   Mix sauce ingredients in large pot. Place over medium heat and cover; bring to a boil, then simmer gently 5 minutes. Add meat balls and heat through thoroughly. Transfer to a fondue pot; serve with toothpicks and cocktail napkins.

Per serving: *Calories:* 207   *Total fat:* 3 grams
% calories from fat: 13   *Carbohydrates:* 17 grams   *Protein:* 30 grams

Wendy & Barb's 4-Layer Dip

This is an easy party dip that takes minutes to make. Serve with low-fat tortilla chips.

1	container Wendy & Barb's "You Won't Believe This Is Low-Fat" Hummus	1
1 cup	Astro non-fat Sour Cream	250 mL
½ cup	President's Choice Mild White Corn & Black Bean Salsa	125 mL
½ cup	Alpine Lace Lite & Lo Cheese, grated	125 mL

Make a bottom layer with Hummus. Add a layer of sour cream. Remove salsa with slotted spoon and add for third layer. Top with grated cheese. Add optional toppings: shredded lettuce, chopped sweet peppers, chopped onion, hot pepper rings, chopped tomatoes.

Per serving: *Calories:* 114   *Total fat:* 2.4 grams
% calories from fat: 18   *Carbohydrates:* 5.8 grams
Protein: 16.9 grams

Vegetable Stock

Mix a batch of this and freeze it in 1-cup (250 mL) portions for future use. It can be used as a substitute for chicken broth or water in most recipes. Makes 8 cups (2 L).

8 cups	cold water	2 L
5	medium carrots, quartered	5
4	medium tomatoes, quartered	4
3	medium onions, quartered	3
3	stalks celery, quartered	3
¼ cup	parsley	60 mL
1	clove garlic, minced	1
½ teaspoon	ground pepper	2.5 mL
½ teaspoon	dried thyme	2.5 mL

Combine ingredients in a 4-quart (3.8 L) saucepan. Boil 1 minute, then cover and simmer 1 hour. Set aside, covered, for 30 minutes. Strain through a fine sieve and refrigerate or freeze.

My Sister's Salsa

Hi, it's Wendy. When my sister Jan and I get together for an hour's worth of girl chat, we make up a batch of this salsa, heat a few low-fat tortillas, mix a pitcher of margaritas, and Olé! We're ready to relax and have fun. Serves 15.

5 cups	Italian tomatoes, peeled and chopped	1.25 L
3 cups	chopped sweet peppers (mixed colors)	750 mL
1 cup	chopped red and white onions	250 mL
1 cup	cucumbers, peeled, seeded and chopped	250 mL
1 cup	cilantro (with stems) finely chopped	250 mL
2	finely chopped garlic buds	2
¾ cup	tomato paste	175 mL
¼ cup	fresh lime juice	60 mL
¼ cup	red wine vinegar	60 mL
½ tablespoon	salt	

Seeded and finely chopped Scotch bonnet peppers: 1 = mild 2 = medium 3 = hot!

Mix thoroughly and enjoy. Store in the refrigerator for up to 2 weeks.

Per serving: *Calories:* 19   *Total fat:* 0.2 grams
% calories from fat: 10   *Carbohydrates:* 4 grams   *Protein:* Trace

My Other Sister's Mexican Spirals

Wendy again. My sister Lori lives in Florida and we've spent many afternoons at the beach with a platter of these Mexican spirals and a cold beer to wash 'em down. The low-fat secret is the Yogo cream cheese (see recipe). Serves 4 (or just Lori and me on a hot day at the beach).

1 cup	firm Yogo cream cheese (see below)	250 mL
¾ cup	Alpine Lace Lo Cheddar Cheese	180 mL
1	diced Jalapeno pepper	1
1	chopped sweet red pepper	1
1	package soft tortillas (large size)	1

Preheat oven to 350°F (175°C). Mix ingredients thoroughly and spread on tortillas. Roll tortillas individually and wrap in plastic film. Refrigerate at least 1 hour. Slice about ¼ inch (1 cm) thick, place on non-stick cookie sheet and bake 20 minutes.

Per serving (6 spirals): *Calories:* 104 *Total fat:* 1.1 grams *% calories from fat:* 10 *Carbohydrates:* 13.8 grams *Protein:* 10 grams

NON-FAT CREAM CHEESE

We call it "Yogo" and it's an ideal non-fat replacement for cream cheese in recipes or on bagels. Start with 2 cups (500 mL) of pure (no fillers like gelatin or tapioca) non-fat yogurt. Pour into a paper coffee filter in the bottom of a colander placed over a bowl. Let stand at room temperature overnight and discard the liquid that gathers in the bowl. Mix with ½ teaspoon (2.5 mL) salt. Store it covered in the refrigerator.

Legal Meatballs

Lean ground turkey substitutes perfectly for high-fat ground beef in this recipe. It's fine for a party buffet. Or serve with low-fat noodles as a main dish for dinner. The meatballs alone can be added to no-fat tomato sauce over pasta. Serves 8 as an appetizer.

1 cup	cooked kasha (buckwheat)	250 mL
1	beaten whole egg or 2 beaten egg whites	1
1 teaspoon	Worcestershire sauce	5 mL
1 teaspoon	grated lemon peel	5 mL
1½ pounds	ground white turkey meat	675 g
2 teaspoons	canola oil	10 mL
1 cup	chicken or turkey broth	250 mL
¼ cup	low-fat yogurt	60 mL
1 tablespoon	cornstarch	15 mL
1 tablespoon	lemon juice	15 mL
1	small carrot, finely shredded	1
1	diced green onion	1

Prepare kasha according to package directions, using chicken-broth variation. Combine kasha, egg, Worcestershire sauce, lemon peel and turkey. Blend well and shape into about 12 balls.

Heat oil in large skillet. Brown turkey balls thoroughly. Add broth, cover and simmer about 20 minutes. Remove cooked balls with a slotted spoon and transfer to a serving platter.

In a small bowl, combine yogurt, cornstarch and lemon juice. Pour into pan juices; heat and stir until sauce thickens. Add carrot and onion; heat and stir several minutes, then pour over turkey balls and serve immediately.

Per serving: *Calories:* 166 *Total fat:* 5 grams
% calories from fat: 27 *Carbohydrates:* 6 grams *Protein:* 24 grams

Chicken-on-a-Stick

For summertime barbecues or winter cocktail parties, these are good beginnings. Serve with spicy peanut sauce and you have satay. Unfortunately, peanut sauce is high in fat, so consider a commercial plum sauce or soy sauce for dipping instead. Try to start these the day before your party—they're best when marinated overnight. This recipe makes 48 toothpick-sized appetizers or 24 skewers.

1 pound	skinless, boneless chicken breasts	450 g
2 tablespoons	cider vinegar	30 mL
2 tablespoons	dry sherry	30 mL
2 tablespoons	liquid honey	30 mL
2 tablespoons	soy sauce	30 mL
2 tablespoons	minced fresh ginger	30 mL
1 teaspoon	sesame oil	5 mL
1 tablespoon	ketchup	15 mL
1 teaspoon	ground coriander	5 mL
2	large minced garlic cloves	2
½ teaspoon	crushed red pepper flakes	2.5 mL
48	toothpicks or 24 wooden skewers	

Cut chicken into thin ½-inch (1.25-cm) wide strips, each 2 to 3 inches (5 to 7.5 cm) long.

Mix thoroughly vinegar, sherry, honey, soy sauce, ginger, oil, ketchup, coriander, garlic and pepper flakes in large bowl. Add chicken strips, stir to coat completely, then cover and refrigerate at least 2 hours (best 8–10 hours).

Soak toothpicks or skewers in water for 30 minutes. Thread chicken onto toothpicks or skewers and broil or grill for 2 minutes on each side or until no longer pink inside.

Per serving (1 skewer): *Calories:* 15   *Total fat:* Trace
% calories from fat: Trace   *Carbohydrates:* 2 grams
Protein: 2 grams

Soups 'n Salads

A Better Borscht

Somebody once said there are as many recipes for borscht as there are Russians. Here's the one that's less than 10 percent fat. It makes a good beginning for a cold-weather dinner, but we like it as a meal in itself, with a couple of slices of pumpernickel bread and some hot tea. Don't overcook the cabbage—steam until just tender. Serves 6.

1 teaspoon	olive oil	5 mL
1	medium onion, finely chopped	1
2	cloves garlic, minced	2
7	medium-sized beets, cooked and sliced.	7
1	14 oz (390 g) can tomatoes	1
1	package beef concentrate and	1
1 cup	water	250 mL
2 tablespoons	cider vinegar	30 mL
1 teaspoon	caraway seed	5 mL
½ teaspoon	salt	2.5 mL
¼ teaspoon	pepper	1 mL
1 cup	cooked shredded cabbage	250 mL
	non-fat yogurt	

"Only the pure of heart can make a good soup."
LUDWIG VON BEETHOVEN

Heat oil in a large sauce pan and sauté onion and garlic until tender. Add remaining ingredients except cabbage and yogurt, and bring to a boil. Simmer 10 minutes, then puree in a blender in small batches until smooth. Return to pot, add cabbage, reheat and simmer another 10 minutes. Pour into bowls and garnish each bowl with a tablespoon or two of yogurt, swirled into the hot soup.

Per serving: *Calories:* 110   *Total fat:* 1 grams
% calories from fat: 8   *Carbohydrates:* 23 grams   *Protein:* 1.6 grams

Low-Fat Vichyssoise

We've always been amused to think that fat, which is hardly elegant, is expected to be a major ingredient in elegant foods—like vichyssoise. Here's a version you'll never have to apologize for, with a total fat content per 10-ounce (300-mL) serving of less than a gram. Enrich the skim milk by adding 1 tablespoon (15 mL) of dry non-fat milk powder to each cup. Serves 6.

The highest form of bliss is living with a certain degree of folly.

ERASMUS

1 teaspoon	canola oil	5 mL
2	large leeks (white part only) finely chopped	2
1	medium onion, finely chopped	1
2	large potatoes, peeled and finely chopped	2
3 cups	skim milk	750 mL
1 cup	vegetable broth	250 mL
½ teaspoon	celery salt	2.5 mL
½ teaspoon	white pepper	2.5 mL
¼ teaspoon	mace	1 mL
½ cup	non-fat sour cream	125 mL
2 tablespoons	chopped parsley	30 mL
¼ cup	chopped green onion	60 mL

Heat oil in large sauce pan. Lightly sauté leeks and onion over medium heat. Add remaining ingredients except non-fat sour cream, parsley and green onion. Bring to a boil and simmer until potatoes are tender.

Remove from heat, cool and separate mixture into two equal parts. Puree one half in a blender, then combine both mixtures. If serving hot, reheat, and swirl in low-fat sour cream just before serving. Pour into bowls. Sprinkle with parsley and green onions. If serving cold, add sour cream prior to pouring into bowls. Garnish as above.

Per serving (1 cup): *Calories:* 125 *Total fat:* .55 grams
% calories from fat: 4 *Carbohydrates:* 28 grams *Protein:* 2 grams

Creamy Asparagus Soup

This is a fine opening course for a small dinner party with friends. But guess what? We lied about the cream! The instant potato flakes add the look and texture of a rich, high-fat cream soup without the fat. Fresh asparagus is preferable, but a 10-ounce (280 g) package of frozen asparagus will work as well, cooked as indicated. Serves 4.

2½ cups	vegetable stock	625 mL
1 pound	fresh asparagus sliced diagonally in 1-inch (2.5-cm) lengths	450 g
½ cup	instant potato flakes	125 mL
1 tablespoon	lemon juice	15 mL
¼ teaspoon	cracked black pepper	1 mL
	dash of salt	
1 tablespoon	minced fresh parsley	15 mL
	thinly sliced lemon	

Combine stock and asparagus in a medium-size saucepan. Cover, bring to a gentle boil, and simmer 3 minutes.

Stir in potato flakes, lemon juice, pepper and salt. Simmer covered for another 2 to 3 minutes, or until asparagus is just tender. Stir in parsley, add lemon slices for garnish and serve.

Per serving: *Calories:* 59 *Total fat:* 1.3 grams
% calories from fat: 20 *Carbohydrates:* 5.9 grams
Protein: 4.6 grams

CLEANING LEEKS

Leeks add a depth of flavor that no other vegetable delivers (in Europe, leeks are often called "The poor man's asparagus"). Leeks need special cleaning, however. To prepare, cut off the roots and almost all of the green top. Then cut in vertical quarters and wash thoroughly in cold water before using.

Basil, Tomato & Green Bean Soup

This is one soup that should be made only in the summertime, when vegetables have their freshest flavor. Also, there is nothing—nothing—like honest-to-goodness fresh basil in a tomato-based meal. You can improve this recipe even more with your own homemade chicken stock, but canned broth or reconstituted stock is almost as good (remember to dilute according to directions). You could even substitute leeks (white portions only, well-cleaned) for the onions. Makes eight 1-cup (250-mL) servings.

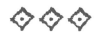

"No man can be a patriot on an empty stomach."
WILLIAM COWPER

2 teaspoons	canola oil	10 mL
2	medium onions, chopped	2
3	medium carrots, chopped	3
2	stalks celery, chopped	2
2	cloves garlic, minced	2
1 pound	fresh green beans, cleaned, trimmed and cut in 1-inch (2.5-cm) lengths	450 g
6 cups	de-fatted chicken stock	1500 mL
½ teaspoon	salt	2.5 mL
¼ teaspoon	pepper	1 mL
3 cups	diced vine-ripened tomatoes	750 mL
¼ cup	fresh basil, finely chopped	60 mL

Heat oil in non-stick pan and sauté onions and carrots for 5 minutes. Transfer to large pot. Add celery, garlic, beans, chicken stock, salt and pepper. Simmer for 20 minutes. Add tomatoes. Simmer for 10 minutes and stir in basil. Serve hot.

Per serving: *Calories:* 87   *Total fat:* 2 grams
% calories from fat: 21   *Carbohydrates:* 12 grams   *Protein:* 6 grams

Santa Fe-Style Couscous

It's so easy to get into a rut with salads if all you change is the dressing. Here's a healthy alternative to lettuce-tomatoes-and-whatever that always reminds us of a summer's evening next to the pool in New Mexico. (It tastes just as good on a winter's evening near the fireplace in Ontario.) Serves 6.

2 tablespoons	olive oil	30 mL
4	green onions, chopped	4
½ cup	sweet red pepper, chopped	125 mL
½ cup	fresh mushrooms, sliced	125 mL
1	large carrot, chopped	1
1	garlic clove, minced	1
2 cups	chicken broth	500 mL
1 teaspoon	ground cumin	5 mL
1 teaspoon	salt	5 mL
¼ teaspoon	pepper	1 mL
	pinch of red pepper flakes	
3 tablespoons	fresh cilantro, chopped	45 mL
1	19 oz (540 mL) can chick-peas, rinsed and drained	1
¾ cup	uncooked couscous	180 mL

In large saucepan, heat oil and sauté green onions, pepper, mushrooms, carrot and garlic for about 2 minutes. Stir in chicken broth spices and cilantro. Add chick-peas, stir well, and bring to a boil. Stir in couscous. Remove from heat, cover and let stand 5 minutes, or until all liquid is absorbed. Chill well and fluff with a fork before serving.

Per serving: *Calories:* 305   *Total fat:* 7 grams
% calories from fat: 21   *Carbohydrates:* 50 grams
Protein: 12 grams

Italian Flag Pasta Salad

The red, green and white colors of this delicious low-fat pasta salad reminded us of the Italian flag—and anything Italian makes us think of great-tasting food! This makes 6 servings and should go nicely with cold roasted chicken breasts (remove the skin!) and crisp white wine.

12 ounces	tricolor rotini	336 g
1	11 oz (310 g) can whole-kernel corn, drained	1
½	sweet red pepper, chopped	½
½	sweet green pepper, chopped	½
1	15 oz (420 g) can kidney beans, rinsed and drained	1
3	green onions, chopped	3
1 cup	no-fat Italian salad dressing	250 mL
2 tablespoons	salad seasonings	30 mL
¼ teaspoon	pepper	1 mL
¾ cup	grated Alpine Lace Lo cheddar cheese	180 mL

Cook rotini according to package directions. Rinse with cold water, drain well, and place in large bowl. Stir in corn, peppers, beans and onions. Mix salad dressing with salad seasonings and add to pasta mixture. Add pepper and cheese and toss. Chill well to blend flavors.

Per serving: *Calories:* 412 *Total fat:* 4 grams
% calories from fat: 9 *Carbohydrates:* 73 grams *Protein:* 17 grams

KING BASIL

According to legend, at one time only kings with golden sickles were permitted to harvest fresh basil. Of all the herbs, fresh basil is the most superior over the dry form. Always try to find fresh basil in season, or consider growing your own. To store fresh basil in the off-season try soaking the leaves in vodka or white wine for several days. Then drain and chop with equal quantities of parsley and seal tightly in jars. Use the mixture spoon-for-spoon wherever fresh basil is called for.

Sesame Chicken Pasta Salad

Sesame has a distinctive nutty flavor everyone loves. This is ideal for buffets or a summer supper. Makes 10 1-cup (250 mL) servings.

3	boneless skinless chicken breasts —about 1½ pounds (700 g) total	3
½ cup	rice vinegar	125 mL
¼ cup	soy sauce	60 mL
3 tablespoons	fresh minced ginger	45 mL
2	garlic cloves, minced	2
1 teaspoon	granulated sugar	5 mL
1 pound	dry small corkscrew noodles	450 g
4	medium carrots, cleaned and julienne-cut	4
2	sweet green peppers, seeded and julienne-cut	2
½ cup	water	125 mL
½ pound	snow peas, washed and trimmed	225 g
½ teaspoon	red pepper flakes	2.5 mL
2 teaspoons	canola oil	10 mL
2 tablespoons	roasted sesame seeds	30 mL

Trim all visible fat from chicken and cut into julienne strips. Combine vinegar, soy sauce, ginger, garlic and sugar in bowl; add chicken. Stir and let stand 30 minutes. Cook pasta in boiling water until firm. Rinse in cold water, drain thoroughly and place in large salad bowl.

Remove chicken from marinade using slotted spoon and cook in non-stick skillet over medium-high heat turning often. Add to pasta.

Stir-fry carrots and peppers in skillet 3 minutes. Add to chicken and pasta. Pour marinade and water into skillet; boil and reduce for 5 minutes. Add snow peas; cook 1 minute, then add to pasta mixture with oil and pepper flakes. Toss well. Serve warm or refrigerate; sprinkle with sesame seeds before serving.

Per serving: *Calories:* 297   *Total fat:* 5 grams
% calories from fat: 15   *Carbohydrates:* 40 grams   *Protein:* 22 grams

The No-Dilly-Dally Potato Salad

We gave it that silly name because, if you say it quickly ten times in a row, it's a great facial exercise.... Actually, it's just to draw attention to the special taste of fresh dill in this dish. Save some sprigs for garnish. Serves 6.

1 pound	red-skinned potatoes	450 g
1 cup	plain non-fat yogurt	250 mL
¼ cup	whole-grain mustard	60 mL
¼ cup	seasoned rice vinegar	60 mL
½ cup	red onion, diced	125 mL
½ cup	celery, diced	125 mL
	fresh ground pepper to taste	
4 tablespoons	fresh dill weed, finely chopped	60 mL

Boil potatoes until tender. Drain, cool and cut into quarters. Blend yogurt and remaining ingredients. Pour over potatoes and mix well. Garnish with whole dill weed.

Per serving: *Calories:* 181   *Total fat:* 1 grams
% calories from fat: 5   *Carbohydrates:* 37 grams   *Protein:* 6 grams

THE SOOTHING HERB

Dill, first used in medieval England, gets its name from the Saxon word "dillan," meaning "to lull" – its reeds were once used to soothe babies to sleep.

Seafood 'n Chili Salad

Proving once again that you don't need butter to enjoy seafood, this makes a fine entrée for a garden party or sit-down dinner. If you prefer, you could serve the veggies raw, tossing them with lemon juice and a teaspoon (5 mL) of caraway seeds. Makes 6 servings.

½ pound	large raw shrimp, shelled and deveined *or* ½ pound large scallops	225 g
½ cup	water	125 mL
¼ cup	lime juice	60 mL
1 teaspoon	canola oil	5 mL
2 tablespoons	minced fresh cilantro	30 mL
2 tablespoons	minced green onion	30 mL
1	dried hapanero chili, rehydrated and finely minced	1
1	clove garlic, finely minced	1
2 cups	shredded green or yellow zucchini	500 mL
2 cups	shredded carrot	500 mL
	wooden skewers soaked in water for 30 minutes	

I am a great eater of beef, and I believe that does harm to my wit.

SIR ANDREW AGUECHEEK, TWELFTH NIGHT (ACT 1, SCENE 3)

Place shrimps or scallops in non-metal dish. Mix water, lime juice, canola oil, cilantro, onion, chili and garlic and pour over seafood. Cover and chill for 2 to 6 hours.

Remove shrimps and scallops, place on skewers, and barbecue or grill until just opaque.

Steam vegetables 3 to 5 minutes and arrange on plates. Remove seafood from skewers and serve atop vegetables.

Per serving: *Calories:* 104 *Total fat:* 2 grams
% calories from fat: 17 *Carbohydrates:* 9 grams *Protein:* 13 grams

Lisa's Raspberry Vinaigrette

Hi, it's Wendy. This recipe came from my friend Lisa Jones, and it proves you don't have to use a lot of oil to enjoy a really good salad dressing. This is wonderful on your favorite greens. Add a few strips of roasted chicken breast to the salad and serve with pita bread and a light white wine or fruit juice for a great summer meal. Makes 6 servings.

2 tablespoons	canola oil	30 mL
1/4 cup	vegetable stock	60 mL
2 tablespoons	raspberry vinegar	30 mL
2 tablespoons	honey	30 mL
1 1/2 tablespoons	Dijon mustard	20 mL
2	cloves garlic, chopped	2
2 tablespoons	skim milk	30 mL
	salt and pepper to taste	

Combine all ingredients in a tightly covered jar or Tupperware container and shake well. Refrigerate until cold—keeps up to one week if refrigerated.

Per serving: *Calories:* 93 *Total fat:* 1.5 grams *% calories from fat:* 14 *Carbohydrates:* 26 grams *Protein:* Trace

I like a cook who smiles out loud when she tastes her own work. Let God worry about your modesty; I want to see your enthusiasm.
ROBERT FARRAR CAPON

Main Courses

Dijon Pork Chops

Butterfly-cut pork chops are generally lean. Avoid excess marbling, and remove all visible fat before cooking. Serve this with "Wendy's Mom's Scalloped Potatoes" (page 197) plus a salad with no-fat dressing for a real "comfort food" meal. Makes 4 servings.

1/4 cup	dry white wine	60 mL
3 tablespoons	soy sauce	45 mL
2 tablespoons	good-quality Dijon mustard	30 mL
2	cloves garlic, minced	2
	pinch of cayenne pepper	
4	pork chops	4

Combine wine, soy sauce, mustard, garlic and cayenne. Cover pork chops and marinate several hours, or overnight, in refrigerator. Broil or barbecue, basting often with marinade, 5–8 minutes per side.

Per serving: *Calories:* 173   *Total fat:* 4.7 grams
% calories from fat: 25   *Carbohydrates:* 1.8 grams   *Protein:* 2.9 grams

Should you have wine with your meals?

Admittedly, it adds calories (but no fat!) and if you have a problem with alcohol, by all means avoid it. But a decent wine adds so much to the enjoyment of a meal. Limit yourself to one or two glasses per meal and choose the best wine you can afford. Then sip it slowly between bites, enjoying the pleasure it adds to the food's flavor. (Many doctors and dietitians believe wine helps digestion too – but we're staying out of that discussion.)

Barb's Never-Tell Chili

Hey, it's Barb. With all the spices working in this chili recipe, you'll never be able to tell it uses turkey instead of beef—which means it's well under 25 percent fat, less than half the normal amount. If you prefer, substitute vegetable broth or water for the wine. Serves 6.

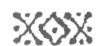

"Cooking is like love—it should be entered into with abandon or not at all."

ANONYMOUS

2 teaspoons	canola oil	10 mL
1	large onion, chopped	1
2	cloves garlic, finely chopped	2
1 pound	ground turkey breast	450 g
¼ cup	parsley, chopped	60 mL
3½ cups	water	875 mL
½ cup	dry red wine	125 mL
2 tablespoons	chili powder	30 mL
¼ teaspoon	chili flakes	1 mL
½ teaspoon	salt	2.5 mL
1 teaspoon	ground cumin	5 mL
1 teaspoon	oregano	5 mL
1	sweet green pepper, chopped	1
1	15 oz (420 g) can red kidney beans, drained	1
1	14 oz (400 g) can tomatoes, with juice	1
1	6 oz (170 g) can tomato paste	1

Heat oil in a Dutch oven; add onion and garlic and cook until onion is tender. Stir in turkey and cook, stirring from time to time, until pink color of turkey is gone. Add remaining ingredients, stirring well. Heat to boiling, then reduce heat, cover and simmer about 45 minutes, stirring occasionally.

Per serving: *Calories:* 230 *Total fat:* 5 grams
% calories from fat: 20 *Carbohydrates:* 29 grams *Protein:* 25 grams

Barb's Mom's "Yes You Can" Ham

Sure you can still enjoy ham on a low-fat diet. Just be sure to choose lean ham, restrict the quantity, and add non-fat ingredients that compliment the flavor of ham. This is a trifle exotic, but very tasty and it's almost a one-dish meal. Serves 4.

4 cups	shredded green cabbage	1 L
1 tablespoon	packed brown sugar	15 mL
1 tablespoon	cider vinegar	15 mL
¼ teaspoon	black pepper	1 mL
½ teaspoon	dry mustard	2.5 mL
1	medium onion, chopped	1
1	large Granny Smith apple, peeled, cored and cut into rings	1
4	extra-lean fully cooked ham steaks —about 3 ounces (84 g) each	4

Place cabbage in non-stick skillet over medium-high heat. Mix sugar, vinegar, pepper, mustard and onion in bowl and stir with cabbage. Add apple rings and cook, stirring frequently, about 5 minutes, or until apple is crisp-tender.

Place ham steaks on cabbage mixture. Reduce heat, cover and cook 10 minutes, or until ham is heated completely.

Per serving: *Calories:* 175   *Total fat:* 5 grams
% calories from fat: 25   *Carbohydrates:* 18 grams   *Protein:* 17 grams

Mixed Herb Lasagna

Serve this to anyone who thinks low-fat vegetarian cooking is dull and boring—it will quickly change their minds! Hint: Make this the night before and store in the refrigerator before baking; the result will be richer and even more flavorful. Serves 6.

1 pound	fresh or dry lasagna noodles	450 g
¼ cup	each fresh parsley, basil and oregano, finely chopped	60 mL
2 cups	low-fat cottage cheese	500 mL
2 ounces	romano cheese, grated	60 mL
4	cloves garlic, minced	4
2 teaspoons	white vinegar	10 mL
2	eggs, lightly beaten	2
4 cups	fresh spinach, washed and dried	1 L
1 cup	tomato sauce	250 mL
1	28 oz (796 mL) can tomatoes	1
1	4 oz (114 mL) can tomato paste	1

Prepare noodles according to package directions (usually boil 4–5 minutes for fresh, 12–15 minutes for dried). Drain and set aside. Combine herbs, cottage cheese, half the romano cheese, garlic, vinegar, eggs and spinach in a large bowl. In a separate bowl, mix tomato sauce, tomatoes and paste.

Coat a 9 × 9 × 2 inch (22.5 × 22.5 × 5.0 cm) baking dish or casserole with non-stick cooking spray. Add a thin layer of tomato mixture (enough to coat bottom of dish. Cover with a layer of noodles, a thin layer of the cheese mixture, another layer of tomato mixture and so on until tomatoes, cheese mixture and noodles are used, ending with a final layer of tomato mixture. Top with remaining romano cheese.

Bake in a 350°F (175°C) oven about 50 minutes, or until bubbling and browned. Let sit 5 minutes before serving.

Per serving: *Calories:* 497   *Total fat:* 10 grams
% calories from fat: 18   *Carbohydrates:* 32 grams   *Protein:* 21 grams

Man-Style Chicken Loaf

What's this thing that men have about meat loaf? We like it too, but traditional meat loaf is unnecessarily high in fat, so we were happy to find this recipe based on chicken instead of ground beef and pork. It's also very good cold, sliced thinly, in sandwiches. Makes 8 servings.

1	egg	1
2	egg whites	2
½ cup	plain low-fat yogurt	125 mL
2 tablespoons	Dijon mustard	30 mL
½ teaspoon	salt	2.5 mL
½ teaspoon	pepper	2.5 mL
1	stalk celery, finely chopped	1
¼ cup	sweet green pepper, finely chopped	60 mL
1	medium-sized onion, finely chopped	1
1	clove garlic, minced	1
1 teaspoon	horseradish (not creamed)	5 mL
2 pounds	ground chicken (white meat only)	900 g
1 cup	dry bread crumbs	250 mL

Combine all ingredients except chicken and bread crumbs in a large bowl and mix thoroughly. Add half the chicken and half the bread crumbs. Blend this portion well, then add the remaining chicken and crumbs. Blend thoroughly.

Place mixture in a non-stick loaf pan, or in a casserole dish sprayed with non-stick cooking spray. Cover loosely with foil and bake at 350°F (175°C) for 1 hour. Remove foil and bake another 20 minutes, or until surface is golden brown. Serve hot or cold.

Per serving: *Calories:* 214   *Total fat:* 5.1 grams
% calories from fat: 22   *Carbohydrates:* 11.8 grams
Protein: 28.6 grams

Berkeley Chicken and Pasta

The sun-dried tomatoes and low-fat content of this dish reminded us of California cuisine—hence the name. Serve with sliced English cucumber sprinkled with chopped green onions and red pepper flakes. And, of course, a chilled California Chardonnay. Serves 4.

¼ cup	chopped sun-dried tomatoes (not oil-packed!)	60 mL
½ cup	vegetable broth	125 mL
4	boneless, skinless chicken breast halves	4
2 tablespoons	dry red wine *or* apple juice	30 mL
2 tablespoons	lemon juice	30 mL
½ cup	sliced fresh mushrooms	125 mL
2 tablespoons	chopped green onions	30 mL
2	cloves garlic, finely chopped	2
1 teaspoon	canola oil	5 mL
½ cup	skim milk	125 mL
2 teaspoons	cornstarch	10 mL
2 teaspoons	fresh basil *or* ½ tsp (2.5 mL) dried basil	10 mL
3 cups	hot cooked fettuccine	750 mL

Mix tomatoes and broth. Let stand at least 30 minutes. Trim fat from chicken.

Pour wine or apple juice into a 10-inch (25-cm) non-stick skillet over medium heat. Add lemon juice, mushrooms, onions and garlic, and sauté 3 minutes until mushrooms are tender. Remove from skillet.

Return skillet to burner and add oil. Cook chicken over medium heat until brown on both sides. Add tomato/broth mixture. Heat to boiling, then reduce heat, cover, and simmer 10 minutes, or until juices from chicken run clear when centers of chicken are pierced. Remove chicken from skillet; keep warm.

Mix milk, cornstarch and basil in small bowl; stir into tomato mixture. Heat to boiling, stirring constantly. Boil and stir 1 minute to thicken, add mushroom mixture, heat through. Set chicken over fettuccine and spoon sauce on each serving.

Per serving: *Calories:* 335   *Total fat:* 9 grams
% calories from fat: 24   *Carbohydrates:* 36 grams   *Protein:* 34 grams

Wendy's Mom's Chicken, Vegetables and Pasta

Chicken and pasta are a great combination for low-fat eating. This recipe is a little adventurous, with endive, radicchio and watercress, but it's rich in both flavor and nutrients. Serves 6.

8 ounces	fresh linguini	225 g
2	large boneless and skinless chicken breasts—about 1 pound (450 g) total	2
½ pound	fresh snow pea pods	225 g
1	medium sized Belgian endive, separated	1
½	small head of radicchio, separated into leaves	½
1	clove garlic	1
2 teaspoons	canola oil (1 + 1)	10 mL
½ pound	bean sprouts	225 g
3 tablespoons	soy sauce	45 mL
3 tablespoons	white vinegar	45 mL
1 tablespoon	prepared mustard	15 mL
1 teaspoon	sugar	5 mL
1	bunch watercress	1

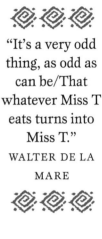

"It's a very odd thing, as odd as can be/That whatever Miss T eats turns into Miss T."

WALTER DE LA MARE

Cook linguini in un-salted water until al dente. Cut chicken in ½-inch (1.25-cm) wide strips. Slice pea pods, endive and radicchio into strips. Slice garlic clove in half. Heat 1 teaspoon (5 mL) oil in non-stick skillet over medium-high heat. Add garlic, cook until golden brown, and discard.

Cook chicken strips in remaining oil until meat loses its pink color throughout. Remove chicken with slotted spoon. Add pea pods and bean sprouts to juices in skillet and toss until tender-crisp. In a cup or small bowl, whisk together soy sauce, vinegar, mustard, sugar and remaining oil.

Arrange endive leaves, radicchio and watercress around rims of 6 plates. Place linguini in center, top first with pea pod mixture then with chicken, and drizzle with soy–mustard vinaigrette.

Per serving: *Calories:* 305 *Total fat:* 6 grams
% calories from fat: 18 *Carbohydrates:* 32 grams *Protein:* 30 grams

High-Brow Tarragon Chicken

Elegant dishes don't always have to be complex, with a list of ingredients as long as a zucchini. Here's an exquisite chicken dish you can serve with boiled small potatoes (toss them with chopped parsley) and sliced fresh tomatoes sprinkled with basil that's as elegant as any—with very low fat content. Banish the children. Light the candles. Cue the Mozart. Serves 4.

4	boneless, skinless chicken breast halves	4
1 cup	dry white wine	250 mL
2 tablespoons	brown sugar	30 mL
1½ tablespoons	grated onion	20 mL
2 tablespoons	soy sauce	30 mL
½ teaspoon	white pepper	2.5 mL
1½ teaspoons	dry tarragon leaves	7.5 mL

Preheat oven to 350°F (175°C). Trim fat from chicken. Mix remaining ingredients in an ungreased rectangular baking dish (about 11 × 7 × 2 inches/27.5 × 17.5 × 5.0 cm). Add chicken, turning several times to coat. Cover and refrigerate 1 hour, turning at least once.

Uncover and bake chicken in marinade about 1 hour; brush chicken in marinade and bake another 15–20 minutes, until juices from thickest part of chicken run clear. Serve immediately, spooning marinade over meat.

Per serving: *Calories:* 170   *Total fat:* 3 grams
% calories from fat: 16   *Carbohydrates:* 9 grams   *Protein:* 27 grams

> ***Don't peel potatoes. Eat the skin, enjoy the flavor, get more roughage... and save time for other things!***

Lemon Sauce Sole

This works well with any mild fish, such as snapper or halibut. Try to use fresh fillets, but frozen fillets will do as well (thaw them well before cooking). By all means, use fresh herbs if possible. Serve this with steamed rice mixed with chopped green onions, and perhaps julienned red, yellow and green sweet peppers stir-fried in a teaspoon (5 mL) of sesame oil. Serves 4.

1 tablespoon	canola oil	15 mL
1 pound	sole fillets	450 g
1 tablespoon	finely chopped onions	15 mL
1 teaspoon	grated lemon rind	5 mL
½ cup	low-fat yogurt	125 mL
2 teaspoons	all-purpose flour	10 mL
1 tablespoon	lemon juice	15 mL
2 tablespoons	chopped fresh parsley	30 mL
1 tablespoon	chopped fresh dill	15 mL
	salt and pepper to taste	

Melt margarine in non-stick skillet over medium heat. Cook fish about 3 minutes on each side, or until opaque. Transfer to hot serving plate.

Add onion and lemon rind to juices in skillet. Cook 1 minute or until onion is tender. Mix yogurt, flour and lemon juice in small bowl, then stir into pan. Add spices, herbs, salt and pepper, stir well and simmer. Return fish fillets to pan, coat with sauce, and serve.

Per serving: *Calories:* 158 *Total fat:* 4 grams
% calories from fat: 23 *Carbohydrates:* 4 grams *Protein:* 24 grams

Harborfront Garlic Shrimp

Shrimp is another good news/bad news food. Good news: It's very low in fat—about 10 percent of its calories. Bad news: It's very high in cholesterol. If your cholesterol level is healthy, enjoy! While a good white Burgundy might be nice with this, we'd prefer a chilled European beer like Beck's or Kronenbourg. Makes 4 servings.

2 teaspoons	canola oil	10 mL
2	large cloves garlic, crushed and finely chopped	2
1 pound	raw, peeled, deveined medium shrimp (thaw if frozen)	450 g
3 cups	sliced fresh mushrooms	750 mL
1 tablespoon	lemon juice	15 mL
	dash of Tabasco sauce	
8–10	green onions, cut in 1-inch (2.5-cm) lengths	8–10
¼ cup	dry white wine	60 mL
2 cups	hot cooked rice	500 mL
	lemon slices	
	parsley sprigs	

Heat oil in heavy skillet over medium-high heat. Cook garlic in oil for 1 minute, stirring frequently. Add shrimp and stir-fry 1 minute.

Add remaining ingredients and stir-fry 2 minutes, or until shrimp are opaque and vegetables are hot. Serve over rice. Garnish with lemon slices and parsley.

Per serving: *Calories:* 255 *Total fat:* 4 grams
% calories from fat: 16 *Carbohydrates:* 27 grams *Protein:* 21 grams

Mushroom-Artichoke Chicken

Another "Boy, is this easy!" recipe. The non-fat yogurt adds a little exotic flavor and fools your palate into thinking it's tasting fat. This would be lovely with rice pilaf and a few cold sliced tomatoes and cucumbers on the side. Serves 6.

1½ cups	sliced mushrooms	375 mL
1½ cups	chicken or vegetable broth	375 mL
1	16 oz (450 g) jar of marinated artichokes	1
6	boneless and skinless chicken breast halves	6
1 cup	plain non-fat yogurt lemon slices	250 mL

The hole in the doughnut is at least digestible.

H. L. MENCKEN

Spray a non-stick skillet with a vegetable-oil coating and sauté mushrooms over medium heat. Remove from pan.

Add broth and marinade from the artichokes. Increase heat and bring liquid to a boil. Add chicken, cover, and poach for 20 minutes, turning chicken occasionally.

Remove chicken and keep warm. Continue boiling liquid until it is reduced by half. Add artichokes and mushrooms, reduce heat and stir in yogurt. Place chicken on heated dishes, spoon sauce over meat, and garnish with lemon slices.

Per serving: *Calories:* 166 *Total fat:* 4 grams
% calories from fat: 22 *Carbohydrates:* 14 grams *Protein:* 19 grams

Curry in a Hurry

We suspect that curry is secretly addictive, but never mind—with fewer than 10 percent calories from fat, you can enjoy as much of this quickly prepared dish as you like. Note: Curry powders vary widely in strength. You may need more or less than shown here, depending on the blend and freshness. Complete the meal with steamed zucchini sprinkled with lemon juice, and perhaps some sliced cucumbers. Serves 4.

Good cuisine is when things taste like themselves.

J. CURNONSKY

½ cup	plain non-fat yogurt	125 mL
½ cup	non-fat mayonnaise	125 mL
3 tablespoons	finely chopped onions	45 mL
1 teaspoon	freshly ground ginger root	5 mL
1 teaspoon	curry powder	5 mL
1 teaspoon	turmeric	5 mL
1 tablespoon	sherry vinegar	15 mL
1 teaspoon	paprika	5 mL
½ teaspoon	ground black pepper	2.5 mL
1 pound	skinless, boneless chicken breasts, cut into ½-inch (1.25-cm) wide strips	450 g
2 cups	hot cooked brown rice	500 mL

Combine yogurt, mayonnaise, onions, ginger, curry, turmeric and vinegar in a small bowl and set aside.

Combine paprika and pepper. Rub into chicken on all sides. Spray a non-stick skillet for 1 second with non-stick spray and place over medium-high heat. Add the chicken and cook 3–4 minutes on each side, until the chicken loses its pink color. Stir in the yogurt mixture. Cook, stirring constantly, for 2 minutes more. Serve over rice.

Per serving: *Calories:* 281 *Total fat:* 2.5 grams
% calories from fat: 8 *Carbohydrates:* 41 grams *Protein:* 23 grams

Saturday-Night Pork Tenderloin

*This is the kind of meal you can look forward to all day Saturday—
then kick back and satisfy a hearty appetite that craves meat. Pork
tenderloin is both lean and tender. Enjoy it more than ever, because
fewer than 20 percent of its calories come from fat. Serves 4.*

1 pound	pork tenderloin	450 g
1	medium carrot, cut in thin 2-inch (5-cm) strips	1
¼ cup	water	60 mL
4	green onions, cut in thin 2-inch (5-cm) strips	4
1 teaspoon	grated ginger root	5 mL
½ teaspoon	minced garlic	2.5 mL
1 cup	orange juice	250 mL
½ teaspoon	grated orange rind	2.5 mL
1 tablespoon	cornstarch	15 mL
1 tablespoon	Worcestershire sauce	15 mL
	pinch of red pepper flakes	
	salt and pepper	

Preheat oven to 350°F (175°C). In roasting pan, roast meat
50 minutes, or until meat thermometer registers 160–170°F
(71–76°C).

About 15 minutes before serving, place carrot strips and water
in a heavy saucepan over medium heat. Bring to a boil, then cover
and simmer for 5 minutes. Add onions, ginger and garlic and
simmer covered for another minute. Combine remaining ingredients
in a bowl and stir into carrot mixture. Cook, stirring constantly
for 2 minutes. Correct the seasoning.

Slice pork thinly and arrange on dinner plates or single large
platter. Spoon sauce over slices.

Per serving: *Calories:* 196 *Total fat:* 4 grams
% calories from fat: 18 *Carbohydrates:* 11 grams *Protein:* 27 grams

Gift-Wrapped Lamb Chops

Save this for a special-occasion dinner when you don't want anyone to know you're eating low-fat—or when you want to brag about how good low-fat meals can be. Parchment paper is available in most large supermarkets and specialty food stores. Steamed baby carrots, a light salad and red wine complete the meal. Serves 4.

½ cup	red wine (Bordeaux or similar)	125 mL
2 tablespoons	finely chopped green onions	30 mL
2 tablespoons	minced fresh parsley	30 mL
2	cloves garlic, minced	2
4	lamb chops cut ¾ inch (2-cm) thick, trimmed of all visible fat	4
4	medium red potatoes, sliced ½ inch (1.25 cm)thick	4
1 cup	thinly sliced mushrooms	250 mL
2 tablespoons	minced fresh dill	30 mL
¼ teaspoon	pepper	1 mL

Preheat oven to 350°F (175°C). Mix wine, onions, parsley and garlic in small bowl. Place chops in large plastic bag. Pour mixture in, shake well, close and refrigerate for 30 minutes, turning occasionally.

Cut parchment into four 1-foot (30-cm) squares. Fold in half and reopen. Place 1 chop on half of each parchment sheet. Top with potatoes, mushrooms dill and pepper. Fold paper over food, seal all edges with a double fold, bring all edges up and twist tightly to hold the folds in place.

Place packets on a cookie sheet and bake for about 20 minutes, or until the paper is browned and puffed. Check doneness by cutting a large X on top of each packet and folding back points. Serve in parchment, garnished with whole dill weed.

Per serving: *Calories:* 138 *Total fat:* 3.3 grams
% calories from fat: 21 *Carbohydrates:* Trace *Protein:* 27 grams

Vegetables & Side Dishes

Wendy's Mom's Scalloped Potatoes

Don't look now, but there's butter in this recipe! We just couldn't help it—scalloped potatoes are a wonderful comfort food, and even with the tablespoon (15 mL) of butter we managed to keep the fat calories below the 30 percent level. Enrich the milk, if you like, by mixing a tablespoon (15 mL) of dried milk powder with the skim. Then enjoy, perhaps with grilled fish or "Dijon Pork Chops" (page 183). Serves 4.

1 tablespoon	butter or canola oil margarine	15 ml
1	large cooking onion, thinly sliced	1
2	large potatoes, thinly sliced	2
2 tablespoons	lemon juice	30 ml
1 teaspoon	thyme	5 ml
½ teaspoon	salt	2.5 ml
1 tablespoon	whole-wheat flour	15 ml
1 cup	skim milk	250 ml
2 tablespoons	bread crumbs	30 ml

Preheat oven to 325°F (160°C). Melt butter in large sauce pan and sauté onion over medium heat until translucent. Add potatoes and mix with onion. Add lemon juice, thyme and salt. Mix well.

Pour half the potato mixture into a lightly greased oven-proof casserole dish and sprinkle with the flour. Add the balance of the potato mixture. Pour milk over entire contents and sprinkle with bread crumbs.

Bake for 1 hour or until potatoes are tender and slightly browned on top.

Per serving: *Calories:* 200 *Total fat:* 3.5 grams
% calories from fat: 16 *Carbohydrates:* 30 grams *Protein:* 12 grams

Educated Baked Potatoes

Why "educated"? Because these potatoes are smart. Instead of soaking up butter or sour cream, they're rich with the flavors of mushrooms, peppers, celery and onion and very low—under 25 percent—in fat. (These could be prepared in advance and frozen for up to a month.) Serves 4.

4	good-sized baking potatoes	4
1 tablespoon	soft margarine	15 mL
½ cup	finely-chopped onion	125 mL
¼ cup	finely-chopped celery	60 mL
2 tablespoons	chopped red or green pepper	30 mL
2 cups	chopped fresh mushrooms	500 mL
¼ cup	chopped fresh parsley	60 mL
¼ cup	skim milk	60 mL
	pinch of cayenne	
½ cup	shredded Alpine Lace Lo Cheddar cheese	125 mL

Preheat oven to 400°F (205°C). Scrub potatoes, prick skins with fork and bake for 50–60 minutes.

Melt margarine in a saucepan over medium heat. Sauté vegetables and mushrooms until tender.

Slice off top of each potato and scoop soft pulp into a bowl. Set the shells aside.

Mash pulp until no lumps appear and add sautéed vegetables and mushrooms plus parsley, milk and cayenne. Add more milk if necessary to produce a thick, creamy texture. Spoon mixture into shells and sprinkle with cheese.

Bake for 10 minutes, or until cheese has melted.

Per serving: *Calories:* 285   *Total fat:* 6 grams
% calories from fat: 19   *Carbohydrates:* 50 grams   *Protein:* 9 grams

Sunset Beets

The combination of rich orange and deep red colors reminds us of a summer sunset. Substitute canned beet slices if necessary.

5	medium beets	5
2	oranges	2
¹⁄₂ cup	orange juice	125 mL
2 tablespoons	water	30 mL
1 teaspoon	cornstarch	5 mL
¹⁄₂ teaspoon	finely chopped chives	2.5 mL
	pinch ground nutmeg	

"Obesity is really
wide-spread."
DAVID GEORGE
BARKER

Trim off leaves and simmer beets in water 35–40 minutes, until tender.

Peel and section the oranges.

Boil orange juice in a small saucepan.

Whisk water and cornstarch together, then slowly whisk into boiling orange juice. Reduce heat and cook until mixture thickens and simmers. Stir one minute more, then add orange sections, chives and nutmeg. Keep warm until ready to serve.

Drain the beets, and slip skins off (if the beets are still hot, hold them with a fork). Slice them about ¹⁄₈ inch (3 mm) thick and arrange on separate serving dishes. Cover with orange sauce and serve.

Per serving: *Calories:* 60   *Total fat:* 0.28 grams
% calories from fat: 4   *Carbohydrates:* 14 grams   *Protein:* Trace

Peas with an Attitude

Peas are fine, but they can be boring. And while fresh peas explode with flavor and nutrition, there comes a time when only frozen are available. This side dish is quick and easy and doesn't depend on the season (except for the fresh spinach, usually available year-round) for enjoyment. Note: *Be careful to include only the yellow part of skin (the zest) when grating lemon. The white pith adds bitterness. Serves 4.*

1	10 oz (280 g) package frozen peas	1
½ cup	frozen small whole onions	125 mL
1 teaspoon	reduced-calorie margarine	15 mL
¼ teaspoon	grated lemon peel	1 mL
1 teaspoon	lemon juice	5 mL
¼ teaspoon	cracked black pepper	1 mL
	pinch of red chili pepper flakes	
2 cups	torn fresh spinach	500 mL

Cook peas and onions in a small saucepan according to package directions. Drain; reserve 1 tablespoon (15 mL) of cooking liquid in saucepan.

Add margarine, lemon peel, lemon juice, pepper and chili flakes to peas and reserved liquid in saucepan. Toss until margarine is melted and vegetables are coated. Stir in spinach. Cover and let stand 1 minute, or until spinach has just begun to wilt.

Per serving: *Calories:* 67 *Total fat:* 0.9 grams
% calories from fat: 11 *Carbohydrates:* 14 grams *Protein:* Trace

Green peas aren't very exciting on their own, but they're fiber-rich. Add them to soups, casseroles, rice, noodles or wherever suitable.

Well-Muscled Brussels Sprouts

You either love or hate Brussels sprouts. We hope you love them, because they are a wonderful source of nutrition and even have strong anti-carcinogenic properties. This is a non-traditional method of serving sprouts (we also like them steamed just so, then sprinkled with lemon juice and sesame seeds) that adds punch to the flavor. Makes 4 servings.

1 pound	Brussels sprouts	450 g
1 cup	beef broth	250 mL
1 tablespoon	Dijon mustard	15 mL
1 tablespoon	minced onion	15 mL
2 teaspoons	lemon juice	10 mL
1 teaspoon	thyme	5 mL
	dash Worcestershire sauce	

"Principles have no force except when one is well fed."
MARK TWAIN

Remove outer leaves of sprouts and cut a small "x" in base of each. Place in a bowl with 3 tablespoons of water and microwave HIGH for 10 minutes, or until tender, *or* steam on stove-top for 10 minutes. (Do not overcook—it brings out a bitterness in this vegetable.) Cover and keep warm.

Combine remaining ingredients in a large skillet over medium heat. Cook 3 minutes, or until mixture is reduced by about one-third.

Add sprouts, toss to coat, and serve immediately.

Per serving: *Calories:* 57 *Total fat:* 0.65 grams
% calories from fat: 9 *Carbohydrates:* 10.6 grams *Protein:* 4.7 grams

Soused Red Cabbage

The ¼ cup (60 mL) of gin is optional (the vast majority of the alcohol is driven off by heat), but it gives the flavor of juniper berries to this spicy sweet-and-sour dish. You can skip the gin entirely, or replace it with 12 crushed, dried juniper berries. This is very good with game or other strong meats. Serves 6.

1 teaspoon	canola oil	5 mL
½ cup	thinly sliced onion	125 mL
1	small red cabbage, cored and cut into 1-inch pieces	1
3	Granny Smith apples, cored, unpeeled and cut into 1-inch (2.5-cm) pieces	3
2 cups	apple juice	500 mL
¼ cup	cider vinegar	60 mL
¼ cup	balsamic vinegar	60 mL
¼ cup	raisins	60 mL
¼ cup	gin	60 mL
1 teaspoon	salt	5 mL
1 teaspoon	cloves, wrapped in cheese cloth	5 mL

Heat oil in large saucepan. Add onions and sauté until tender. Add remaining ingredients except cloves. Mix well. Bring mixture to boil. Add cloves in cheesecloth, cover and simmer 45 minutes. Remove lid, take out cloves, raise heat, and boil until just enough liquid remains to keep cabbage moist. Serve hot.

Per serving: *Calories:* 187   *Total fat:* 3.2 grams
% calories from fat: 15   *Carbohydrates:* 37 grams   *Protein:* 2 grams

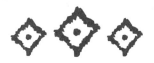

Desserts & Other Rewards

Peppermint—Chocolate Angel Cake

Gee, is low-fat eating ever tough, huh? This is virtually fat-free, yet still tastes a little decadent, thanks to the peppermint–chocolate flavor. Frozen fruit or preserves can substitute for fresh. Serves 12.

12	egg whites	12
¾ cup	sifted pastry flour	180 g
¼ cup	unsweetened cocoa powder	60 g
1 teaspoon	cream of tartar	5 mL
1 teaspoon	peppermint extract	5 mL
½ cup	honey	125 mL
	icing sugar	
	fresh fruit—strawberries,	
	raspberries, blueberries or peaches	

Preheat oven to 350°F (175°C). Let egg whites stand at room temperature in a large bowl for 30 minutes. Sift flour and cocoa powder together 4 times.

Beat egg whites with a mixer on high speed until foamy. Add cream of tartar and peppermint extract. Beat on medium speed until soft peaks form. Slowly add honey while continuing to beat mixture until stiff peaks form. Sift one-quarter of flour–cocoa mixture over eggs and fold in gently. Repeat sifting and folding one-quarter of flour and cocoa at a time until finished.

Spoon batter into an ungreased 10-inch (25-cm) Angel Food pan (or "tube pan") with removable bottom. Using a thin knife, slice through batter to remove air pockets.

Bake for 30 to 35 minutes, or until cake springs back when lightly touched. Cool on wire rack. Remove from pan and dust lightly with icing sugar. Slice and serve with fresh fruit.

Per serving: *Calories:* 121   *Total fat:* 0.6 grams
% calories from fat: 4   *Carbohydrates:* 26 grams   *Protein:* 2 grams

Wendy's Florida Lime Pie

You can't eat out in Florida without spotting Key Lime pie on the menu. I love limes, but pie pastry is a no-no in a low-fat diet. So I was happy to come across this recipe using meringue as a crust instead of a topping. It's tart, light and luscious! Makes 8 servings.

Crust:

2	egg whites	2
¼ teaspoon	cream of tartar	1 mL
½ cup	granulated sugar	125 mL

Filling:

2	egg yolks	2
4	egg whites	4
¾ cup	water	180 mL
⅔ cup	granulated sugar	170 mL
1 tablespoon	grated lime rind	15 mL
⅓ cup	fresh lime juice	1
1	envelope unflavored gelatin	80 mL

Preheat oven to 275°F (135°C). Beat egg whites and cream of tartar with electric mixer until soft peaks form. Gradually add sugar and continue beating until stiff. Spread meringue on foil-lined 9-inch (22.5-cm) pie plate, raising edges about 1 inch (2.5 cm) above sides. Bake about 1 hour (meringue should be light gold in color). Remove foil carefully.

Whisk egg yolks separately in non-aluminum saucepan. Gradually add water, half the sugar, and lime rind. Cook over low heat, stirring constantly, 10 to 15 minutes until mixture thickens slightly. Remove from heat.

Sprinkle lime juice with gelatin and let stand 2 minutes. Stir gelatin mixture into eggs; cover and refrigerate 10 minutes. Beat egg whites (4) until peaks form. Continue beating while adding remaining sugar until stiff and fold into lime mixture. Spoon into meringue shell and refrigerate until set. Serve cold.

Per serving: *Calories:* 146   *Total fat:* 1 grams
% calories from fat: 6   *Carbohydrates:* 31 grams   *Protein:* 4 grams

Bravo Biscotti

Most hard cookies such as ginger snaps are lower in fat than soft cookies. This recipe for delicious twice-baked Italian cookies manages to bring the fat content down even lower, to less than 1 gram per cookie, thanks to the use of egg whites and a minimum amount of oil. Great for coffee breaks! Makes about 40 cookies.

3 cups	all-purpose flour	750 mL
½ cup	cornmeal	125 mL
2 teaspoons	baking powder	30 mL
	pinch of ground cinnamon	
3	lightly beaten egg whites	3
½ cup	honey	125 mL
2 teaspoons	canola oil	10 mL
1 teaspoon	almond extract	5 mL
½ cup	lemon juice	125 mL

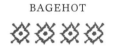

The greatest pleasure in life is doing what other people say you cannot do.

WALTER BAGEHOT

Preheat oven to 350°F (175°C). Blend flour, cornmeal, baking powder and cinnamon. In a separate large bowl, mix egg whites, honey, oil and almond extract.

Whisk the flour mixture into the egg mixture, and add enough lemon juice to form an easily handled dough.

Divide dough in half, and form each portion into a roll about 12 inches (30 cm) long. Line a cookie sheet with parchment paper. Place rolls about 6 inches (15 cm) apart on the paper and press down on each roll until it is 1/2 inch (1.25 cm) high.

Bake for 35 to 40 minutes. Remove from oven, cool slightly, then cut each into ½ inch (1.25 cm) slices. Places slices, cut side down, on cookie sheet and bake on one side until golden brown (about 10–15 minutes). Turn over and bake until golden brown on other side. Cool on wire rack and store in air-tight container.

Per serving (1 cookie):   *Calories:* 58   *Total fat:* 0.8 grams
% calories from fat: 5   *Carbohydrates:* 13 grams   *Protein:* 1 grams

Three-Generation Oat Cookies

All kids love cookies. So do their grandparents. These are tasty enough—and low enough in fat—that adults can enjoy them as well, which just about covers everyone. This makes about 3 dozen.

A good hostess is like a swimming duck – calm and unruffled on the surface and paddling like hell underneath.

ANONYMOUS

1²/₃ cups	rolled oats	325 mL
1 cup	all-purpose flour	250 mL
1 teaspoon	baking powder	5 mL
1 teaspoon	cinnamon	5 mL
¹/₂ teaspoon	baking soda	2.5 mL
2	egg whites	2
³/₄ cup	brown sugar	185 mL
¹/₄ cup	corn syrup	60 mL
¹/₄ cup	skim milk	60 mL
1 teaspoon	vanilla	5 mL
1 cup	raisins	250 mL
1 cup	chopped dried apricots	250 mL

In a large bowl, combine oats, flour, baking powder, cinnamon and baking soda. In a second bowl, beat egg whites lightly and blend with sugar, syrup, milk and vanilla. Add to oat–flour mixture, stirring until all ingredients are moist and dough is thick. Stir in raisins and apricots. Drop by spoonfuls onto non-stick cookie sheet and bake at 375°F (190°C) for 12–15 minutes or until set and gold in color. Allow to cool before serving.

Per serving (1 cookie):   *Calories:* 76   *Total fat:* 0.3 grams
% calories from fat: 4   *Carbohydrates:* 18 grams   *Protein:* 1.5 grams

Luscious Orange Bavarian

This is almost sinfully rich, yet each serving has barely a trace of fat and less than 100 calories total! It's also light, making it the perfect end to a multi-course dinner. If serving to guests, make it the day before and refrigerate in attractive ½-cup (125-mL) serving dishes, perhaps garnished with mint and orange or tangerine sections. Makes 8 servings.

1	envelope unflavored gelatin	1
1 cup	fresh orange juice	250 mL
½ cup	low-fat yogurt	125 mL
	grated rind of 1 orange	
½ teaspoon	vanilla	2.5 mL
2	egg whites	2
½ cup	granulated sugar	125 mL
¼ cup	skim milk	60 mL

Sprinkle gelatin over orange juice in top of double boiler. Set aside for 5 minutes, or until gelatin has softened. Heat contents over simmering water until gelatin dissolves. Refrigerate until mixture is syrupy.

Stir yogurt, orange rind and vanilla into mixture until smooth.

In separate bowl, beat egg whites until soft peaks form. Gradually add sugar while continuing to beat until peaks are stiff.

In another bowl, beat skim milk until it is frothy and at least doubled in volume.

Fold, first, egg whites, then milk, into orange mixture. Spoon into dishes and refrigerate at least 2 hours until set.

Per serving (½ cup):   *Calories:* 87   *Total fat:* Trace
% calories from fat: Trace   *Carbohydrates:* 18 grams
Protein: 3 grams

FORGETTING FAT

We want everyone to enjoy their food as much as we do. If you miss certain flavors in your foods because you've eliminated fat, replace them with herbs and spices. Be prepared to experiment a little. Not all your experiments may work, but we'll bet you discover new ways to stimulate your appetite and still lower your fat intake.

Here's a primer on herbs and spices we enjoy, and some dishes you might try them in:

★ **BASIL**—Wonderful on tomatoes and corn.

★ **BAY LEAVES**—Not just for soups and stews but in any dish with beans or beets. Be sure to remove before serving.

★ **CARAWAY SEEDS**—Powerful little guys (so use sparingly) that add zest to cabbage and turnip.

★ **CAYENNE**—Another powerhouse. Try a pinch wherever you'd like an extra "bite" of flavor.

★ **CILANTRO**—Chop and use like parsley with beans, corn and curry dishes. Also called coriander.

★ **CELERY SEED**—Gives new flavor to salads, salad dressings and soups.

★ **CHIVES**—For a delicate onion-like flavor in light sauces.

★ **CLOVES**—Try a dash in tomato sauce for pasta, and add one or two to fresh fruit dishes.

★ **CUMIN**—Great for beans and curry dishes.

★ **CURRY**—Actually a mixture of several spices. Some love it, others aren't so sure.

★ **DILL WEED**—It's a wonderful fresh herb with almost any vegetable, but especially, cucumbers, potatoes, carrots and cabbage.

★ **GARLIC**—Frankly, we like garlic in almost everything but desserts! Always use fresh cloves, stored in a container that permits air circulation. Avoid garlic powders and garlic salt.

★ **GINGER**—Another wonderful spice. Just cut a fresh ginger root, inhale the aroma, and see if your taste buds don't get excited! Terrific when grated and combined with garlic.

★ **NUTMEG**—It's not used in enough dishes, in our opinion. Try nutmeg on spinach, parsnips, carrots, Brussels sprouts and broccoli.

★ **PAPRIKA**—Mostly for color on potato salads or in Hungarian dishes.

★ **PARSLEY**—Fresh parsley is mild and enhances other flavors. Add it as a garnish too.

★ **ROSEMARY**—A lovely summer-style spice that's fine in salads and soups as well as on potatoes, green beans and peas.

★ **SAGE**—Careful with this one. It's a fine herb but can overpower other flavors.

★ **SAVORY**—Experiment with it in potato dishes, cabbage, beans, soups and casseroles.

★ **TARRAGON**—Another classic you should always have on hand. Add it to beets or almost any vegetable, as well as sauces and salads.

★ **THYME**—A hearty herb for soups and stews.

CHAPTER ELEVEN

Get Started—
Walking, Jogging
and Weight-Training

Most people have two ideas about exercising for fitness. The first idea is that it must be strenuous to be beneficial. They assume that unless you are huffing and puffing during and immediately after exercising, it's not doing you much good. Actually, you should be able to carry on a conversation while performing any exercise activity (with the exception of competitive events such as marathons); if the activity leaves you too short of breath to speak, tone it down.

The second wrong idea is that exercise is both hard work and boring. Correction: It *can* be hard work and boring if you let it. But it can also be relaxing, interesting and exciting, if you prefer. In fact, if you find any exercise that is both too hard and too boring, either change your activity level or stop it. But go find another one as quickly as you can—one that promises to keep you interested.

If you've never succeeded in maintaining an effective exercise program, you probably need some rules or guidelines to follow. This is especially appealing if you choose not to join an organized aerobics program—one of those weekly events where a large number of overweight people in the back of the room do what one perfectly sculpted person in the front of the room tells them to do. We're not opposed to aerobics classes, but we think they're a little like giving ten dollars to charity so you don't feel guilty about all the underprivileged people in the world. Spending an hour or so a week in an aerobics class shouldn't be the end of your exercise program—it should be the beginning.

The most effective exercise programs are the ones that you develop, choose and follow for yourself. Then you can ensure they match your schedule, your needs and your abilities, and help you enjoy 100 percent of the satisfaction.

So here are "Wendy and Barb's Ten Suggestions for Exercise Activity." Unlike the Ten Commandments, following them faithfully doesn't guarantee you a place in heaven. But we can promise an improvement in your body weight, muscle tone and overall health if you combine them with our low-fat eating guide.

1. *There are no rules.* Or, to put it more accurately: *The only rules worth following in an exercise program are the ones you set for yourself.* Remember that no one else in the entire universe is exactly like you. Your body has unique abilities and activity needs, and you have your own social, career and family concerns. It's important for you to control your own life, and having someone barking at you, either from the front of the gym or through your TV speaker, is not much fun. We think that's one reason many people don't succeed at exercise programs. Still, common sense tells you some things you should do before getting started.

They include:

★ *Seek some medical advice.* Have your physician confirm that your heart can stand the strain of a certain level of physical activity, and that you don't have any special dietary needs.

★ *Start slowly.* You didn't gain all that weight in a week, or even a month, and you can't expect to lose it that quickly.

★ *Try to be consistent.* "Consistent" doesn't mean boring or obsessive. It means that you'll honestly try to follow a planned routine, and that missing one day of your routine isn't enough for you to give up completely. Discover things you like to do which reflect, as closely as possible, the guidelines in Rule #2, below. Remember that quantity substitutes for quality; if you can't jog half an hour every other day, walk for an hour each day. If you'd rather play tennis than jog, play tennis as often as you can. In fact, the best all-round exercise program is probably a "Mix 'n Match" schedule. You might walk 40 minutes for three days a week, jog for 20 or 25 minutes two days a week and play tennis or racquetball on weekends.

It may work for you.

Many people find that exercising just before their evening meal actually reduces their appetite level and they eat less dinner. They balance it by eating larger breakfasts the next morning. That's not so bad— an old proverb goes:

Eat breakfast like a king.
Eat lunch like a prince.
Eat dinner like a pauper.

If you find that exercising before dinner reduces your appetite for a heavy evening meal and helps you load up on juice, fruit and grains the next morning instead, stay with it.

2. *Choose an activity that keeps your legs and buttocks busy.* This is where your body's largest muscles are found, and anything that keeps them moving burns maximum amounts of energy. Doing arm-curls with weights or push-ups from the floor is fine for upper-body muscle tone. But real progress is made when you use your legs and buttocks.

3. *Make it a continuous activity instead of a stop-and-go exercise.* Walking for 3 miles (5 kilometers) non-stop is far more effective than walking the same distance but stopping to chat with friends every few blocks. The idea is to get your heart rate up and keep it up for a period of time.

4. *Start with too easy rather than too hard.* When some people begin an exercise program, they throw themselves into it as though training for the Iron Man Triathlon. That's a mistake. First, if you're out of shape, you could severely damage your body. Second, it's going to be painful, and when you don't see immediate visible improvement—and you almost certainly won't—you'll say "What's the use?" and give up. Third, it's unnecessary—even if you're exercising at only two-thirds of your body's ability, your cardiovascular system will still benefit from it, and you'll eventually be performing more strenuous activities with less effort: in other words, you'll become fit!

Hey, It's Wendy

We always stress that you should work out your own fitness schedule, depending on the time available, obligations to family and work, whether you're a "morning" or a "night" person, and so many other things. But people at our seminars, and those who approach us with questions about fitness, always seem to be interested in what we do to keep fit. So here's my schedule:

Monday	Weight training (using a small set in my bedroom or a larger set in my rec room) or visiting a local gym: 30–40 minutes
Tuesday	Running for 30 minutes (in bad weather I use a StairMaster or go to the gym)
Wednesday	Weight training: 30–40 minutes
Thursday	Running: 30 minutes
Friday	Weight training: 30–40 minutes
Saturday	OFF
Sunday	Family activities: biking, hiking, roller-blading, etc.

5. *Avoid fit friends during exercise.* Working out with fit friends when you're just getting started is like attending your first choir practice with Luciano Pavarotti—you'll be either inspired or discouraged, and we'd put our money on the latter. By pushing you too fast, too far and too often, fit friends can make you feel inadequate—or, even worse, cause injury. If you believe companionship may help you succeed, find someone who is at the same level as you are. If it helps, compete against each other for progress.

6. *It doesn't matter how far or how fast you go.* Exercise by time, not by distance. When exercising by time, all you need is a wristwatch, and you can go anywhere you want instead of sticking to a fixed—and eventually boring—route. Also, you won't be tempted to push yourself too hard "just to get it over with."

7. *Think about anything you want when exercising— except calories.* Sure, you can measure how many calories you've burned with an exercise. But go beyond that. *The key benefit of exercise is not just that it burns calories, but that it changes your body chemistry.* Remember all that stuff about carbohydrates and muscle cells? Go back and read it over again, if necessary. Instead of visualizing all those faceless calories being burned in your body, picture your muscle cells growing larger and more efficient—that's your real goal.

8. *Eat often.* This is the good-news side of exercise that few people think about. When you begin your exercise program, don't skip meals on the assumption that you'll lose weight faster. Eat foods that are higher in complex carbohydrates, like fruits, vegetables, grains and beans, and eat smaller quantities several times during the day. Why? Because out-of-shape people need higher levels of blood sugar to help consume fat in their bodies. It's very important to keep your metabolism balanced when on a fitness program. Eating too little will slow your metabolism and make becoming fit a more difficult challenge.

9. *Don't let weather be an excuse for not exercising.* Okay, it's a cold, rainy day in November and you'd rather curl up with a good book and a cup of hot tea than venture outside. We understand. So dangle a carrot in front of your nose (not literally, unless that works for you!): promise yourself a hot bubble bath if you'll finish a brisk 40-minute walk on this miserable day. Or go mall-walking if there's one nearby. Or slap a Bob Marley or corny disco tape on the CD-player and dance for half an hour.

10. *This isn't Sunday school—perfect attendance doesn't win you points.* If you skip a day now and then, so what? Everybody does. Just get back to it when you can and don't assume you're a failure. Most of all, never call yourself "lazy" or "hopeless." You're neither—you're a human being. You're a miracle of evolution and design; you are not, never were, and never will be perfect. But if you get back to your exercise routine tomorrow, you'll soon be darn good! (Note: If you become a runner or weight lifter, your body needs time off now and then—especially at the beginning. Just be sure to get back at it.)

MAKING THE SHOE FIT.

Since comfort is a prime consideration when getting ready to exercise, be sure to find the most comfortable shoe available. Here's a hint: Many athletic-shoe manufacturers make women's workout shoes narrower in the front than men's. If you find your workout shoes are too tight across the toes, walk across the store and try on some men's styles.

Get started walking!

The best way to get started on a physical-activity program is simply to rise up out of your chair, step outside, and walk. Walk through your neighborhood and look at the trees, the sky and the gardens, if you're in the suburbs. Walk in a park during the day—nod and smile to passersby, *but keep walking*. Walk with a friend or your partner, chatting and gossiping as you go, *and keep walking*. Walk during your noon-hour lunch break. When you want a change of scenery, especially on spring and fall weekends, drive to the country, park your car well off the road, and set out facing traffic; walk about 30 minutes in one direction, then turn around and walk back to your car.

Don't underestimate the advantages of walking: It needs no special training, uses those heavy muscles in your thighs and buttocks, requires little in the way of special clothes or equipment, and is not likely to result in any physical damage if you use common sense while doing it.

In fact, we believe that the best kind of regular exercise for most people is a combination of walking and weight lifting. You might even consider altering the two—walking one day for 45 minutes to an hour, and lifting weights the next day for 30 minutes or so.

Of course, there are right ways and wrong ways to do anything—and that includes starting and maintaining a walking program. So here are some tips from us and from some experts in the field we've listened to:

1. *Put your best foot forward.* It almost goes without saying that the most important investment you can make is in your shoes. Cheap canvas shoes or your favorite old gardening sneakers just won't do the job. You don't have to invest in hundred-dollar-plus professional athletic shoes that look as complex as the innards of a computer. In fact, shoes designed for certain sports such as tennis and basketball are generally not suitable for extended periods of walking. So avoid them, and go shopping for quality name-brand shoes designed specifically for walking. It's best to choose a sports specialty store, for wide selection and staff with lots of product knowledge and fitting skill. *Hint:* Try on shoes at the end of the day when your feet are slightly larger than normal. Wear workout socks, and don't forget that one foot is probably larger than the other, so try both shoes on for size.

When choosing shoe brands and models, look for these features:

★ If you have a pair of old sneakers or similar shoes, bring them with you. Show them to the sales person, who should be able to determine your walking style (Hard on the heels? Favor one side over the other? Scuffing the toes? Need strong side support?) and choose the brand and model that suits you best.

★ Always ask to see three or four different brands or styles, covering as wide a price range as possible. The most expensive shoe may not provide the best performance, so don't assume you always have to pay top dollar.

★ Test the sole. It should be both durable and flexible. Some walking shoes have soles shaped like rocking-chair runners—rounded from heel to toe for a natural rolling motion when you walk. You may prefer this shape, or your walking gait may not be suitable for it. Try pairs with flat or rounded sole shapes and see for yourself.

★ Examine the heel bottom. It should be wide for extra stability when you walk. Narrow heels will be more difficult to wear for extended periods.

★ Look inside the heel at the "counter." This is the area that grips the back of your foot, holding the shoe in place as you walk. A poor fit here can cause pain, early fatigue and severe blisters. Make sure the counter holds your foot without binding or slipping.

★ The upper materials should be breathable, which means either leather or a special synthetic mesh.

★ The inside tip of the shoe should be about $\frac{1}{2}$-inch (1.25 cm) longer than your longest toe, enabling your toes to spread as they walk.

★ Buy for comfort, not style. Style won't mean a thing when you're 2 miles from home with blisters the size of bottlecaps on your feet.

Hi, It's Wendy

Barb and I started a walking group, just to encourage people who attended our seminars to get out and enjoy some activity. We would meet every Sunday, and week by week the group grew until we looked like a small migration!

When we first talked about walking 3 miles (5 km) non-stop, a lot of people would tell us they couldn't go that far. "Yes, you can," we'd say. "Just walk slower if you have to." Eventually a lot of those slow walkers became fast walkers, and soon they became runners—people who didn't believe they could walk 3 miles were running that distance and more!

It occurred to me that there was a real lesson here. Whenever someone now says, "I don't think I'm capable of that," I answer: "Surprise yourself—I did!"

It may take a friend or spouse for support, it may take joining a club—but whatever it takes, tell yourself that you're going to surprise yourself with your own determination and ability, and I bet you do!

2. *Dress for the occasion.* In cold weather, dress in layers so you can trap body heat when you need it, and cool off as your temperature rises. And always wear a hat, preferably with a brim. It shields you from the sun in summer, keeps you dry in the rain, and helps retain body heat in winter.

3. *Take something with you.* A friend is nice, of course. Just be sure you can both maintain the same pace and distance, or one will suffer from overexertion while the other is bored from insufficient exercise. An apple or other non-fat snack is good as a reward at the halfway mark. Portable tape recorders and radios? They're fine, but pay attention to where you're walking when wearing them, especially on city streets. Some walkers just like to take their own thoughts with them; walking lets your mind play with a problem or idea, and many walkers we know start out with a problem and come home with a solution.

4. Start out right. If you haven't walked long distances at a steady pace, begin with 30-minute walks. Increase your pace, but maintain your time as you feel yourself growing more fit. Then extend your time by 10 or 15 minutes and relax your pace again. Another suggestion: When getting started, vary your walking pace from time to time. For example, walk briskly for a city block or two, then slow down for another block. Your body will tell you the pace it prefers.

5. Walk proudly. Also known as "Listen to your mother," because these tips sound like the kinds of things your mother might have told you:

★ **Hold your head high,** keep your back straight and walk with a confident attitude. Walking's not for wimps.

★ **Pull in your tummy as you walk.** It's great for those lazy muscles.

★ **Swing your arms as you walk.** Try keeping your elbows bent at a 90-degree angle.

★ **Find your natural stride.** Make it as long and as powerful on the push-off as you can and still feel comfortable.

★ **Listen to your feet.** If you hear "thump-thump" as you walk, you're either taking strides that are too long, or you're lifting your knees too high. When walking correctly, there should be almost no sound at all from your feet.

★ **Listen to your lungs too.** They should be working harder than normal without straining; you should be able to carry on a conversation as you walk.

★ **Reach for the stars.** Every ten minutes or so while you're walking, lift your hands over your head and stretch hard.

★ **Don't avoid hills.** Moderate hill-climbing as you walk really builds stamina and strength—many trainers feel hill-climbing separated by long periods on level ground is more effective than wearing weights on your ankles and wrists.

★ *Choose several routes.* Discover five or six places where you enjoy walking, so you can avoid boredom. Look for interesting locations such as alongside a lake or the seaside, or through a wooded conservation area.

★ *Be careful out there.* Use common sense where and when you walk. Try to walk during the day, when you can be seen easily. If walking at night, wear light-colored or luminous clothing, walk in well-lit areas, and take a friend.

Quantity is better than quality.

Some sports and activities are considered less effective in raising your fitness level than others. Tennis and swimming, for example, are not nearly as good at burning calories and toning muscle as most of their advocates think. But if you do enough of any activity that uses a wide range of muscle groups, you'll benefit. For example, if you spend 4 or 5 hours gardening—turning over earth, bending and lifting, walking back and forth—chances are your body will benefit in many ways as much as from a 30-minute run.
The idea is to get active and stay active!

Get started running.

Walking should be your basic exercise. For many people, it may be the only one they either need or can do with safety. But don't discount running or jogging; much more efficient ways to burn calories, improve cardiovascular performance and raise HDLs (remember those high-density lipoproteins that are so good at scouring cholesterol from your arteries?).

Running versus Jogging:

What's the difference? People who care about these things say that if you can do better than 1 mile (1.6 km) in 8 minutes, you're running. If it takes longer than 8 minutes to travel that distance, you're jogging.

Running is not just walking at a faster pace. It's a much different kind of body motion, demanding its own equipment, style and environment.

1. *Use different shoes for walking and running.* The basics of choosing a dealer and getting the proper fit hold true for both walking and running footwear. But proper running shoes are designed differently from walking shoes. Running places much higher stress on your feet, ankles, legs and spine. Without a proper running shoe, all of this continuous pounding can cause injury, especially at the beginning, when your weight may be a little high and your style marks a little low. Also, if you know where you'll be doing most of your running—on asphalt, grass, concrete, bare ground or a track—tell the sales person; that way, you'll be looking at shoes whose wear characteristics are appropriate for the surface.

Most of all, look for comfort, support and cushioning to help the shoe absorb all that punishment before it reaches your body.

Hello, It's Barb

All running shoes are not created equal! Start by looking in the phone book for a store that specializes in running shoes and athletic equipment.

At the store, insist that they check your shoe size and analyze your gait. Don't settle for the first pair of shoes you try on—try on several different shoes and compare how they feel. Then ask for a guarantee. Any reputable store that takes the time to fit you with a shoe will stand behind it if you have problems. After all, if they recommended the shoe for you, it's not your fault—it's theirs.

2. *Dress a little lighter.* You'll be building up much more body heat, so consider loose comfortable shorts and a cotton T-shirt in summer. In winter, add layers of clothing you can tie around your waist or carry in your hand as you get warmer.

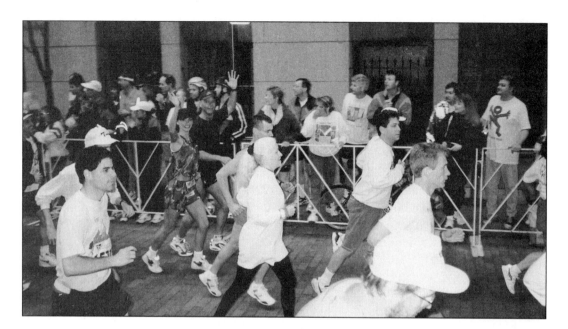

After more than 26 miles (40 km), when I finished my first marathon, I finally left behind the woman in the picture on page 79. (She's still back at the start line somewhere, enjoying a strawberry shake with fries…)

3. ***Dress in style.*** You'll be much more conspicuous when running than walking. So if people are looking at you anyway, you might as well dress yourself up a little. Choose an outfit that flatters you and makes you feel good. No, it won't get you in shape faster, but if it makes you feel better about yourself and gets you out more often, you'll enjoy the same benefits. Don't spend a fortune (unless you have it!); just take a little more care in fit and color.

4. ***Get prepared.*** Running places much higher stress levels on your body, especially the large muscles of your legs. Don't begin any extended or high-speed running without first taking a few minutes for a whole body stretch and warm-up. (This is a good rule for any exercise.) Here are some basic stretches to perform; do each three or four times before setting out:

★ *For your lower back:* Stand with back straight, looking forward. Raise one leg, grasp it firmly just below the knee, and pull gently but firmly toward your chest. Hold for a count of three. Repeat with other leg.

★ *For the back of your thighs:* Bend one leg slightly and thrust the other forward, resting on the heel. Lean slightly forward, resting your hands just above the knee of your back leg. Gently try raising your hips (you should feel the muscles on the back of your bent leg tighten). Hold for a count of three. Repeat with other leg.

★ *For the front of your thighs:* Support yourself with one hand on a post or wall; keep your back straight and your head up, looking forward. Keeping your knees together, bend one leg and reach behind you with your free hand to grasp the ankle. Lift leg as far as you comfortably can and hold for a count of three. Repeat with other leg.

★ *For your calves:* With your back straight, place one foot a stride ahead of the other. Keeping the heel of your back foot on the ground, rest your hands on your leg above the knee and lean forward, bending the knee of your forward leg, until you feel tightness in the calf of your back leg. Hold for a count of three. Repeat with other leg.

5. *Choose your course.* Running demands a smoother, more predictable course than walking, so avoid hazards such as traffic, pedestrians, kids on skateboards and mothers pushing strollers.

Running on grass or firm sand along a waterfront is wonderful, but to be more realistic you'll probably be running on bare ground or asphalt.

Wendy Here to Talk about Running

I enjoy running, even though I keep a slow, close-to-the-ground pace (those darn arthritic knees!). Interesting thing: After I encouraged Barb to eat low-fat and get fit, she came back and talked me into entering my first competitive race—a local 3-mile (5 km) event to raise money for the Arthritis Society. Was that appropriate or what? Anyway, I finished the race, and there was nothing more satisfying. Here I was, an arthritis sufferer from childhood, running 3 miles to raise money that will be used to fight that disease!

6. *Develop your technique*. Keep your back comfortably straight as you run, with your head up and your shoulders relaxed; leaning forward can cause painful shin splints and back problems. Don't clench your fists, but bend your arms to a comfortable position.

There are as many different running techniques as there are runners, and all work well to one extent or another. To find your own style, try "floating" over the ground as you run. This means running with minimum impact force and with equal-length strides. When you're "floating," it's as though you are riding atop your legs while they do the work, smoothly and effortlessly beneath you. Here's another way of thinking about it:

There's a difference between playing the piano and playing music. When you begin running, you'll be playing the piano; when you're "floating," you're playing music.

7. *Follow a program*. Like lifting weights, running requires time to develop both a safe technique and a proper level of fitness. Do not rush yourself into a running program, or your body will never forgive you. Think of it as a romance—it's better to start out slowly with your eyes open, aiming for the long term, than to plunge into things with a "What the hell!" attitude.

We doubt that anyone ever gave you a program for developing and maintaining a romance, but here's one for building your running and fitness activity. We suggest you spend at least one week at each level if you've been fairly active and are under age 45; two weeks at each level if you're under 45 and not active; three weeks at each level if you're over 45.

GETTING STARTED (Running & Walking)

Level 1	Level 2	Level 3
3 times weekly: run 1 minute, walk 30 seconds. Repeat 10 times.	4 times weekly: run 3 minutes, walk 1 minute. Repeat 6 times.	4 times weekly: run 5 minutes, walk 1 minute. Repeat 5 times.
Level 4	**Level 5**	**Level 6**
5 times weekly: run 10 minutes, walk 2 minutes. Repeat 3 times.	5 times weekly: run 10 minutes, walk 1 minute. Repeat 3 times.	5 times weekly: run 30 minutes, no walking

It's all right to vary your activity. Most trainers agree that your body will achieve higher fitness levels more effectively if you vary the level of intensity, especially when you reach Level 6. If you run hard one day, use the next day for extended walking, or set yourself a more leisurely pace. This enables your body to respond better to exertion and should help prevent injury.

Beyond Level 6, consider Fun Runs. Setting off on a weekend run with a few hundred other souls can honestly be fun. It's both a social event and a workout, and the competition can give your energy a boost (but unless you're in peak condition, run for the enjoyment of it, not for the prize at the end).

Listen to Your Heart[1]

Wear a wristwatch with a second hand or indicator when exercising, and periodically check your pulse rate (beats per minute) to ensure it's within the safe range. To calculate your safe pulse range, as recommended by the American College of Sports Medicine (ACSM), use the following formula (write your figures in the appropriate areas, as indicated):

Basic rate (everyone starts here):   **220**

Subtract your age (write it here):   ____

This is your maximum heart rate: ____

Multiply this by 0.55 =   ____

(This is the low end of your range.)

Multiple your maximum by 0.9 =   ____

(This is the high end of your range.)

Example: If you're 40 years old, 220 − 40 = 180

180 × 0.55 = 99 = low end of pulse rate

180 × 0.9 = 162 = high end of pulse rate

HINT: *Count your pulse for 10 seconds and multiply by 6 to obtain beats-per-minute without standing around for 60 seconds. If it's too high, slow down your activity; if it's too low, speed things up a bit.*

---

[1]Of course, anyone with a record of heart problems should exercise only under the direction of a qualified medical professional, and we advise everyone over the age of 30 to have a medical examination prior to launching a fitness program.

Hi, It's Barb

We keep saying that everyone has to work out her own schedule, but I know it's always interesting to see how other people balance their fitness needs with the rest of their life. So here's mine. I like cross-training, because it never gets boring to me. Here's what my typical week looks like:

Monday	Run 30 minutes with my husband, Brian
Tuesday	Run 30 minutes
Wednesday	Bike at least 45 minutes with our son, Jake
Thursday	Swim 45 minutes
Friday	My day off!
Saturday	Run 45 minutes
Sunday	Bike with Jake and Brian: 45 minutes

Plus do weight training for 10 to 15 minutes about three days a week. When Brian and I do our run together on Monday, we talk and plan our week. My twice-weekly biking sessions include Jake strapped in his seat behind me. He gets fresh air and new scenery, and I get the benefit of pedaling an extra 30 pounds around town. Thanks, Jake!

My twice-weekly running sessions may be alone or with some friends, and our Sunday biking trips may take the whole day if we head for a park or stop for lunch.

Get started lifting

True weight training needs a gym setting and a professional trainer to guide you in developing basic techniques and setting a program to help achieve a realistic objective. And if you're using weight training to strengthen specific joints or muscle groups, especially for rehabilitation purposes, a physiotherapist is a must.

But sweaty gyms are unattractive to many people—not to mention a drain on your budget. And most people, men and women alike, are most interested in strengthening and adding tone to their upper body and abdominal muscles. For these, a few simple exercises and some logical precautions are all that's required. Just remember to always warm up first, and look ahead to a full program of weight lifting exercise to develop your body symmetrically.

Weights made easy (and cheap).

It's not necessary to invest in metal weights, especially if you're just getting started. Raid your recycling bin for plastic jugs - the kind used for milk or other liquids. Look for two identical containers, fill them half or more full of water or sand (if getting started, make the weights no heavier than 3 pounds or 1.5 kg), and you're on your way. As you grow stronger, add more water or sand to increase the weight.

Wendy (foreground) demonstrates the tricep "kick-back," which firms the back of your upper arms. Barb is doing "curls," which add tone to your bicep area (the front of your upper arm).

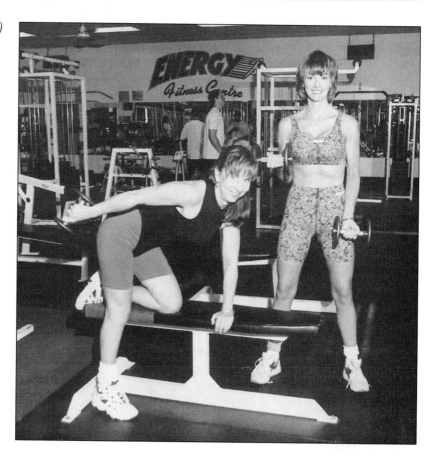

1. *Strengthening and toning your upper arms.* You need to work on two muscles here: your *biceps* (on top) and your *triceps* (underneath).

For biceps (these are called "curls"):

- Stand erect, feet about shoulder-width apart, knees slightly bent.
- Holding a weight in each hand with arms down, keep your elbows close to the body.
- Lift one weight to your shoulder.
- Lower and repeat with other arm.
- Repeat 10 times with each weight. Rest for a minute and repeat 10 times again.

For triceps (this exercise is known as a "tricep kick-back"):

- Support one knee on a bench or chair; slightly bend the other leg, keeping the foot flat on the floor.
- Steady yourself with a free hand.
- Your back should be straight and your eyes forward.
- The arm holding the weight should be bent, with the elbow tucked in.
- Extend the arm backwards; hold and return.
- Repeat 10 times. Change arms and repeat. Rest for a minute and repeat 10 times with each arm.

Hi, It's Wendy

When I joined a gym a few years ago, determined to strengthen my body by working out, the gym was divided into two sections: Male and Female. The Female room was primarily for aerobics—women moving and dancing to music—with a few Nautilus machines here and there.

But the Male room had *weights*, and the word was that weights would turn women into muscle-rippling, masculine-looking people who, for all we knew, might start growing beards and repairing pick-up trucks.

Well, the more I read about fitness and the more I talked to women like me who felt that weight training could be part of their workout, the more intriguing it became. So a group of us began lifting weights—in my case, to both build overall strength and relieve the pain I was suffering from arthritis.

Weight training is *not* a threat to your femininity, and it's not a fad either. It's an honest-to-goodness way to "round out" your fitness program, help shape your body, and add an inner feeling of power and accomplishment that no other activity can equal. I hope you'll try it.

2. *Chest muscles.* This is the only non-surgical method known to increase your bust size! Muscles called pectorals support the breasts; increasing their size and tightening their tone literally lifts and extends the chest wall. (Who needs a WonderBra?) The weight-lifter's term for these exercises is "flyes."

● Lie on a flat bench. Bending your knees, place your feet flat on the bench—or, if you prefer, on the floor on either side of the bench.

● Extend your arms, weights in your hand, elbows slightly bent.

● Slowly raise your arms above your chest until your hands are almost touching. Hold and slowly lower again, controlling the weights precisely at all times.

● Repeat 10 times. Rest 1 minute and repeat again.

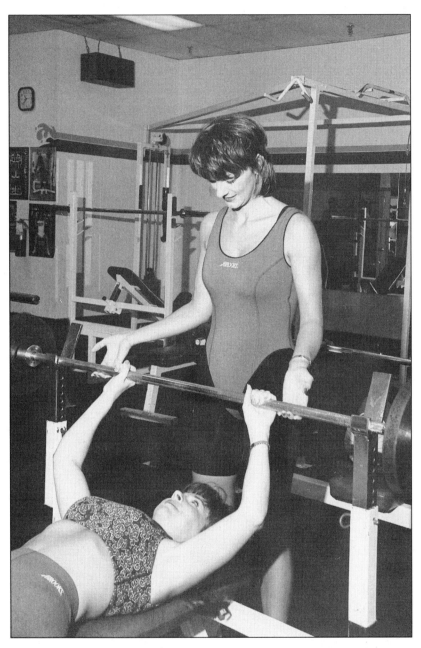

Almost every woman can benefit from improving her pectoral muscles. It's an ideal way to "reduce" your waist by expanding your chest. Have someone experienced in weight training get you started, then set yourself a long-term target such as lifting (or "pressing") your own weight.

Wendy Again

When Barb and I do our seminars, I always avoid the term "body-building" because that creates some of those obsolete ideas I referred to earlier—you know, where women visualize their head on Arnold Schwarzenegger's body? So I use terms like "strength-training" or "resistance exercises."

Many women attempt to reduce their thighs with leg lifts—lying on their sides and raising one leg in the air until their toes point to the ceiling. Have you tried those? Didn't work, did they? That's because it doesn't strengthen the major muscles in your legs—the quadriceps on the top of your thighs, and the hamstrings, running up the backs of your thighs. When you're doing leg-lifts, these big guys are just loafing!

Squats get your quads and hamstrings working, burning fat and pulling into shape. Take it from me—I once had a classic pear-shaped body, and I hate pears! Squats made the biggest difference in shaping my thighs and reducing my hips. And my body's my own—not Arnie's.

Anyway, here's what I do during weight training:

10-minute warm-up (stretching)
Monday: Work on triceps and chest
Wednesday: Work on back and biceps
Friday: Work on legs (quadriceps and hamstrings)
                       and shoulders

A couple of other suggestions:
   Do ab crunches (sit-ups) whenever and as often as possible—
       at night, before going to bed, works for me.
   I have a chin-up bar in my bedroom doorway—great for
       shoulders and pecs!
   I do calf raises at the gym or on my stairs.

3. *Buttocks and upper legs.* In case you're wondering, these muscle groups are known as the *gluteus maximus* (your buttocks), *quadriceps* (front of upper legs) and *hamstrings*

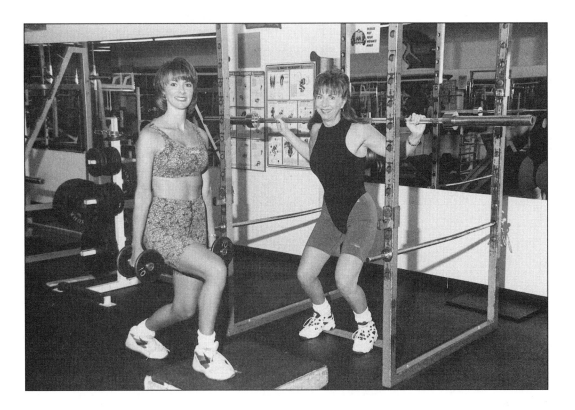

(back of upper legs). The technical term for these exercises is "squats."

- Stand upright, back straight, eyes forward, feet about shoulder-width apart and knees slightly bent.

- Keep your arms close to your body, hands lightly grasping weights.

- Keeping your feet flat on the ground, slowly lower your body until your thighs are about parallel with the ground. Hold for a count of three and raise yourself again to a standing position.

- Repeat 10 times. Rest 1 minute and repeat again.

For your legs, try "lunges," as Barb (foreground) demonstrates, and "squats," as Wendy is doing with the weight across her shoulders.

It's Wendy Again

Everyone who begins lifting weights thinks in terms of shaping his or her body, and that's the ultimate goal, of course. But something soon happens *inside* after you've been lifting weights for a few weeks—something that's just as good, in its own way.

First, you begin to think of food as fuel. You grow aware of the way different foods can affect your performance while lifting weights, and how important protein and complex carbohydrates are to your body.

Next (don't laugh), you start having conversations with your body—positive conversations, not the negative things it used to tell you when you walked past a mirror and wondered who that unattractive person was staring back at you. These conversations go something like:

Upper arms: "Got a lot of extra strength here."

Shoulders: "Let's try some chin-ups—things are a little flabby."

Legs: "Okay, we're ready to lift another 10 pounds any time you are."

You start *listening* to your body, and it tells you positive things.

Finally, the inner change is a sense of independence and confidence that nothing else can give you. Your body isn't just something handy to carry your head around on—it's a finely tuned, well-running machine that you're proud of, and that you won't let anyone or anything mess with again.

4. *Shoulders.* These are called "lateral raises" and exercise the main muscles in your shoulders, called "deltoids."

• Stand upright, feet about shoulder width apart and knees slightly bent.

• Hold one weight lightly in one hand; keep free arm behind your back.

• Raise the arm with the weight to shoulder height, palm facing down. Hold for a count of three, then slowly lower again.

• Repeat 10 times with each arm. Rest 1 minute and repeat again.

5. *Abdominal muscles.* We're talking about your stomach muscles here. Physical fitness types call them "abs" and doctors refer to them as *rectus abdominis* muscles (the ones that get that washboard effect on hard bodies) and *intercostals*, muscles on the side of your tummy. Whatever you call them, (we'll say "abs"), you need strong ones to show a flat tummy to the world.

The best way to strengthen these muscle groups is by doing "crunches," and here's how to get it done:

• Lie on your back, supporting your head with your fingers. Relax your knees, bending them slightly, and cross your ankles.

• Using your abdominals, curl your shoulders and your upper back slightly off the floor. Hold this contraction for a count of three, then slow return to your start position.

• Repeat this motion several times. While performing the exercise, try twisting from side to side; you'll feel your intercostal muscles tighten as you do.

• For a variation of this exercise, bend your knees up until your feet are flat on the floor.

6. *Back muscles.* Many people complain about back pain. The truth is, sore backs are almost always weak backs—often made weak from carrying around too much excess weight! And, by the way, here's one thought for the day: Instead of starving yourself to make your waist look thinner, why not feed yourself well and make your upper back larger? The visual effect will be the same and your physical well-being will be so much better!

This series of routines will develop width in your upper back; combine them with routines for chest and shoulders described above, and you'll actually sculpt your body shape from the inside out!

• Grasp the lat bar, arch your back and keep it arched throughout this series of motions.

• Using your back muscles, pull the bar down until it touches your upper chest at the base of your neck.

• Keeping your elbows back, slowly and smoothly return to the start point. Repeat this entire motion 10 times, rest 1 minute, and repeat the series again.

Once you've started weight training, check for results that make you feel productive. Squeeze your biceps after performing the curl exercise. Feel that hardness? That's tight muscle tone. Grip your thighs after doing a series of squats. Notice how they're not as loose as before? Take satisfaction in the changes you can feel, and you'll soon notice changes you can see.

If you choose to get started with the simple weight-training exercises listed above, maintain the number for about two weeks, performing the exercises every other day. Then double the number for another two weeks. After a month, add some weight—no more than 2 pounds (1 kg)—and begin with the basic number of exercises, doubling them again after a month.

Wendy, One More Time about Weight Training

Remember that gym I told you about? Two years after three others and myself began insisting on weight training, the owner had to double the size of the Co-ed weight room. Today, women of all ages, sizes and physical condition (some in wheelchairs, some having suffered heart attacks or strokes) are there every day, strengthening their bodies with weights.

So you don't have to be a pioneer. You just have to want a tighter, more sleek and efficient body badly enough.

CHAPTER TWELVE

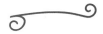

Keep Going with Other Activities

Too many people have this image of themselves living in Lycra and dining on yogurt. Well, we don't do either. As you probably know by now. We follow two guidelines above all else:

1. Use "cruise control" to keep fat calories under 25 percent of total.

2. Find things we enjoy doing that keep our muscles from imitating Jell-O.

The second point covers walking, jogging and weight training, because they're most effective at burning calories and shaping our bodies. Other activities aren't quite as effective, but find time for them anyway. Better still, at least try them—you may discover a new hobby that leads to new activity that leads, finally, to an almost-new you!

True or False Questions and Answers.

There are many misconceptions about fitness, usually held by people who are less than fit (to be kind). Here are some we've gathered, along with answers from various expert sources:

★ "The best time to exercise is first thing in the morning."

False! It may be fine for some people, but most will benefit more from exercise around 5:00 P.M.

★ "You should see results from diet and exercise after about a week."

False! It takes about a month for real lasting change to happen.

★ "Exercising the same body part every day is best."

False! Alternate body parts to get the most from exercise.

★ "Building strong muscles is hard on the bones."

False! Additional muscle tissue strengthens bones and helps prevent osteoporosis.

★ "Proper breathing is important during a workout."

True! Never hold your breath during exertion, such as lifting weights.

★ "The body burns most of its fat during the first 20 minutes of exercise."

False! Your body tends to burn little fat at all in the first 20 minutes; most fat is consumed after that time.

★ "Set yourself the goal of looking like professional models on TV and in magazines."

False! Fewer than 20 percent of people have body shapes that match those of professional models. Aim instead for good all-round physical shape and an ideal weight range.

★ "If you're more than 30 percent over your ideal weight, you should exercise after eating."

False! You'll burn more calories by working out before a meal and watching your food intake when you eat. If you're within 30 percent of your ideal weight, you should work out after eating, however.

Hiking—A natural extension of walking.

Unless you live among mountain trails, this probably isn't an activity you can perform several times a week. But it's a fine fitness activity because it works out your body while restoring your soul. Another good tip: Even if the only time you manage to go hiking is on weekends, if you enjoy it sufficiently—and most people love it!—that's an extra reason to walk on weekdays and keep yourself in shape.

★ You'll need some special equipment for longer hikes. Properly designed hiking boots (extra cushioning, ankle support, waterproofing, sturdy sole that grips the ground) and walking socks (they act like wicks to transfer moisture from your feet to the air) are important. Shorts or slacks with extra pockets to hold camera, binoculars, maps are handy as well.

Swimming—Fun and generally safe but . . .

Swimmers don't like to hear this, but their favorite activity isn't as beneficial to their health as most think. In his book *Fit or Fat,*[1] Covert Bailey points out that, of the thousands of people he has tested for body fat, swimmers always carry more fat than runners or cyclists. He notes that mammals who spend their lives in water, such as seals and walruses, have bodies that are literally wrapped in blubber—not good role models!

In spite of that, even Covert Bailey agrees that swimming can be a good starting point for overweight people who are just beginning an exercise program. It's also ideal for anyone with muscle injury, back problems or join disorders.

---

[1](Boston: Houghton Mifflin, 1991).

Hi, It's Barb

I try to swim for about 45 minutes or 1 mile (1.6 km). I vary every length I swim—one length of breast stroke, one length of front crawl. A couple of suggestions: First, never look at the clock on the wall while you're swimming. This is one sport that seems to take longer to do than others, and if you glance at the clock now and then you'll think you're swimming forever—or at least to Europe. Also, try to avoid swimming at family times; it's difficult to concentrate on your stroke if you're dodging young children or water toys.

★ You will, of course, need access to a pool (lakes and oceans aren't best to maintain full intensity while swimming).

★ Even if you consider yourself a good swimmer, have yourself evaluated by a swimming coach to ensure your stroke is correct; incorrect techniques or an ineffective stroke will reduce the benefits of exercise.

★ Consider aqua-aerobics. It's a relatively new form of pool activity; since it takes place in the shallow end of the pool, you don't even have to know how to swim to join in!

Hey, It's Wendy

How about roller-blading?

When my son was fifteen, I'd drive him to the local school track and sit there in the car, mesmerized by the sight of him gliding so gracefully around the track on his roller-blades. I'd also watch him "grabbing air" on skate boards and snow boards, envying his energy and his willingness to risk injury just to enjoy a sport he loved and to exercise his body.

Maybe it was the new confidence I'd acquired from weight training. Whatever it was, one day I realized how roller-blading was a great fitness sport. It works out those big leg muscles and gets your cardiovascular system going. Best of all, I'd get a good workout without jarring my weak knees, the way jogging can. Hey, all I had to do was conquer my fear.

And I did. I got fitted for roller-blades by a sports-equipment professional, received some guidance from my boyfriend, listened to words of advice from my son ("Stay near the grassy area. Expect to fall a few times. Trust your equipment.") and I was off.

I love roller-blading now. It was another excuse to buy a new outfit (a cute roller-blading one) and something else for my sister Lori and I to do when I visit her in Florida. Unlike my son, I keep the wheels planted firmly on the ground.

Roller-blading has its risks, of course. You can expect to pick up minor scrapes and bruises while you're learning. But it's one of those activities you'll love doing, and it won't seem like exercise at all—even though it's a really good one!

This is obviously posed, because nobody has to coax Wendy to go roller-blading— not since her son, Lee (right), first convinced her to try it. It's fun and a great workout. Just use common sense, wear protective gear and get started!

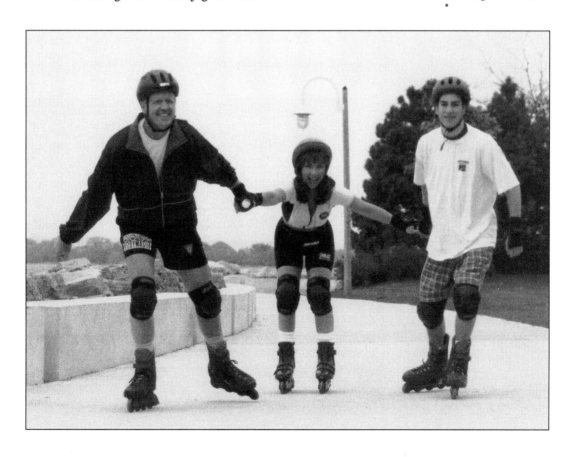

Cycling—The one you may almost overdo!

An open road, a mild day and a good bicycle. Set out in the morning and you may not want to return until nightfall. That's how many people view cycling. Even better, it's an excellent fitness activity for leg, back and shoulder muscles too. And, if you discount the risk of collisions and accidents, cycling is less likely to cause injury to joints and muscles than running or other strenuous activity.

The drawbacks? You can (but don't have to) spend thousands of dollars on your bicycle. Road hazards, both moving and stationary, have to be considered. And weather plays greater havoc on cyclists than on walkers or runners. We think cycling should be a part of everyone's physical-activity program, if only to serve as a break between sessions of walking and jogging.

Physical activity doesn't have to mean sweat and strain. It can be as much fun as a family bicycle ride, as Barb, Brian and Jake demonstrate. The secret is to eat low-fat and stay as active as you can.

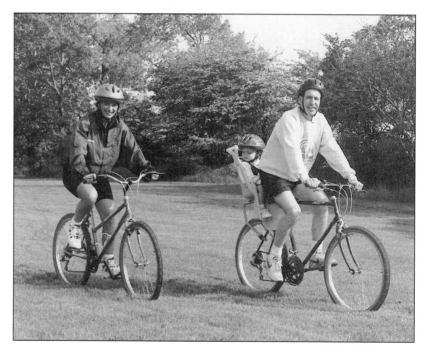

Hi, Barb Here

Cycling is great with young kids because they can ride along behind you. Be sure to find them a safe, sturdy seat and approved helmet, of course. When Jake isn't with me, I get a bit adventurous—I climb hills, which really works the quads (those big muscles on top of your thighs), and zoom down the other side. When my husband is riding with me, we find open areas of the road to race each other. It's a great way to get fresh air and a good workout, and feel like a kid again!

★ Cycling is good aerobic exercise, but since you use fewer muscles (none of them weight-bearing), you'll have to cycle twice as long as jogging to obtain the same benefit. The good news—you probably won't mind!

★ Cycling out of doors on a two-wheeler is preferable to using a stationary bicycle indoors because you work out more muscles just keeping your balance.

★ Don't go overboard choosing a bicycle unless you're in the fortunate position of not being restricted by your budget. You can pay from $200 to $5,000 for a bicycle, but you'll ride both the same way. When choosing a bicycle for fun and fitness (as opposed to competition and status), follow these steps:

1. Go to a specialist. It's worth paying an extra few dollars at a cycle shop, if only for help in finding the correct bicycle size and design.

2. Ask about used bicycles—you could save a bundle.

3. Look for a recreational or hybrid design—it's more stable than a racing bike and lighter than a mountain bike.

4. Choose a men's style—the crossbar adds stability and makes the bicycle easier to pedal.

5. Fitting a bicycle should be like fitting a shoe. Select one that feels good and ride around a little before deciding.

★ A helmet is an unfortunate necessity; in some states and provinces, it's also a legal one.

★ When cycling, try to maintain a pedal speed of about 55 to 60 revolutions per minute at the beginning. As your fitness improves, bump this up to about 70 rpm.

Cross-country skiing—Now you're talking fitness!

Nothing burns fat faster than cross-country skiing. The injury rate is low, and the start-up costs are reasonable—you can be on the snow for $100 or less! You see as much scenery as you do when cycling, and the whole family can join in. Wow, what a sport!

All right, there are some drawbacks. First, it's a winter activity, which turns some people off right away. More important, you really should be moderately fit, because cross-country skiing demands good arm/leg coordination and balance.

★ Rental equipment is available for those just starting out.

★ As with jogging, dress in layers when skiing cross-country; you'll build up a lot of body heat with this one.

★ Never leave a marked cross-country trail if skiing alone.

★ Indoor ski machines (you've seen them in the TV commercials) are expensive and often gathering dust within a few weeks of purchase. If you really want one, haunt the used-sporting-equipment stores for a bargain.

Racquet sports—more fun than exercise?

Will playing tennis, squash, racquetball and badminton make you fit? The answer seems to be a definite "maybe." One fitness experts says playing squash twice a week will improve your fitness level; another points out that your body will benefit as much from 15 minutes of jogging as it does from 1 hour of tennis.

The drawback of racquet sports seems to be that they're classified as "stop and go" activities, along with downhill skiing, football and calisthenics. True aerobic activity requires steady motion for a minimum of 12 minutes.

Our suggestion? Play a racquet sport for fun and for a good general workout. But to make yourself lean, mean and *Armed and Dangerous*, try extended walking, running or cycling.

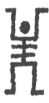

CHAPTER THIRTEEN

But Enough about Us....

We started out to become *Armed and Dangerous* to save ourselves—or at least our self-esteem. But once we began sharing all we learned and all we had done, many people told us we were really on to something.

It's always nice to have someone else confirm that your ideas work for them as well as they work for you. And it's a wonderful feeling when you can literally change other people's lives for the better. We've seen it happen, and many of the women who have attended our seminars and our grocery-shopping tours have become our friends.

We asked a few of them to share their experiences with us and with you. So here they are. See what you learn from them. Try becoming *Armed and Dangerous* yourself. When you succeed, write us. (Hey, we're not going to stop at one book, and we'll be looking for all the stories we can find for the next one!)

Tracy's story:

"For years I thought a belt was an alcoholic drink!"

Tracy came to one of our earliest seminars with a sense of humor and a determination to lose weight. At 5 feet, 10 inches, she weighed 230 pounds, fitted into a size 24 dress and was told she carried her weight well—a phrase she hated!

The effects of her excessive weight were heightened by a problem with weak knees ("You know—the kinds that run in the family . . .") and back problems, which she blamed on her mattress. This was bad enough, but Tracy also suffered from more serious and more deeply entrenched problems too.

> I had anxiety attacks and symptoms of menopause at age 37. I often laughed at myself, but now I see that it was just a form of defense against pain. Like swimming pools with waterslides—I'd have to go down them sideways because I was too wide to fit in one normally, and then I'd laugh with the kids in the pool when I'd hit the water like a beached whale and create a tidal wave!

Tracy saw an advertisement promoting our seminars and decided to attend. Even then, being overweight had an influence on her attendance. First, she found two friends to bring with her ("Being overweight took away my self-esteem, so I never did anything alone"), and she had to buy a new outfit ("If I was to be the biggest person there, I was going to look the most fashionable. Some fashion—elastic-waist shorts with a long matching blouse to hide my tummy . . .").

Never mind—she was there, she listened, she believed and she began:

> I couldn't get past the fact that Barb has lost 60 pounds in just five months! I kept telling my friends that if I worked as hard as she did, I could look like her by Christmas. I wanted Wendy and Barb to take me home and teach me their secrets. I wanted to say "I'll clean, you cook, we'll eat and I'll lose." But I didn't—I just listened and wrote notes like crazy. Then I went home and babbled to my husband about understanding how fat works on your body and how to eat better, and especially how to lose this weight. My husband's response was "Look out, world—my wife is on a mission!" And I was!

Tracy went shopping the next day, armed with new knowledge about fat content. What was normally a half-hour chore became a two-hour voyage of discovery as she studied and began to understand all the data on food packages. She learned even more on one of our accompanied supermarket tours and was so enthusiastic that we invited her to join our Sunday 3-mile (5 km) walk-and-jog group.

When Tracy discovered she could run a full 6 miles (10 km), she raised her target higher and began entering races. She hasn't won a race yet, but she has won prizes and finished every race she has entered. In fact, we were so impressed with Tracy's accomplishments that we asked her to model clothes for one of our televised fashion shows.

> I was 35 pounds lighter than when I began, and I modeled a jumpsuit with a belt on it. What a thrill! For years, I thought a belt was an alcoholic drink! My dress size has changed to a size 13, and I'm working toward a size 11. When I reach that goal, I'm going to reward myself with a matching satin bra and panty set. My self-esteem improves with every pound of fat or inch of waistline I lose—and which I forbid to ever return! So far I've shed 42 pounds, and I'm aiming to lose another 15.

Pretty good stuff, huh? Tracy's well into weight-training and looks terrific. But the change inside her is just as dramatic and important as the change to her weight and figure:

> I tolerated who I was before, but now I love who I am today. I like being me! I like trying on new clothes from stores where only my friends could shop at one time (I'd have to go down the street to the Big 'n Tall shops). Listen, here's a hint when you start to shed your weight—if you think it's not worth the effort to keep going, wear an old, bigger-sized dress for a while and see if that isn't motivation enough!

We still keep in touch with Tracy, and whenever one of us calls and her husband answers, he thanks us for helping to make his wife more active, mobile and healthy. He probably agrees with the newest goal Tracy has set for herself: "I want to feel as good as Demi Moore looks!"

Corinne's story:
"There is a way to fit running into my schedule ... which is my time!"

Sometimes we think that the first lesson to be learned in becoming *Armed and Dangerous* is to be selfish. We mean it in a nice way, of course. But most women (and a good portion of men, we'll admit) are raised with the idea that it's better to give than to receive. It's a nice thought and makes everyone feel warm and fuzzy inside, but there are times when we think it was invented by a department-store sales manager as a Christmas slogan.

Being selfish isn't a matter of either giving or receiving. It's a matter of loving yourself in every sense of the word—of realizing that, if you are unable to love yourself, you're not very well equipped to love anybody else at all.

We still believe in giving to others. It's giving *in* to others that we think raises a problem with many women. That's where many of us, in our opinion, could stand to be a little more focused on our needs first.

Corinne is a good example. You would hardly call her selfish; "busy" would be a better description. She's a working mother who attended one of our seminars and, as she put it in her letter to us, "saw the light" on low-fat eating. She also began running on a regular basis—something she hadn't done since her high-school days.

> Running has brought me new challenges and a feeling of great satisfaction for myself! My life is busy raising two small children, working, and taking care of household obligations. But if there's a will, there's a way to fit running into my schedule ... which is *my* time. With much delight, I completed an 11-mile (18 km) run last December. It was a challenge for me but I did it! *My next dream is to complete a marathon!*

Corrine pointed out to us something we see over and over again in women who begin eating low-fat foods and launching their own wellness program: They notice benefits they never expected. Sure, they finally begin losing weight permanently. They fit into clothes they would never have dared to wear before. And they have more energy, too.

But something else changes inside. With Corrine it was this: "I feel better now than I ever have. My moods and depression and my binge eating are all under control. . . ."

We're not psychologists. Heck, we're not even nutritionists! But it's pretty obvious to us that a lot of so-called emotional problems are directly related to physical condition in more ways than anyone may really understand.

That's why we get impatient with people (and there are fewer of them every day, thank goodness!) who almost defend the idea of being overweight by saying that we're promoting attractive appearance as much as anything else.

So what's wrong with that?

Why not change the things you can, especially when so many other benefits are waiting for you to enjoy—benefits like a longer, more active life; a generally better feeling of well-being; better defense against a whole range of serious, debilitating diseases; and, here it comes: a chance to wear clothes you haven't dreamed of wearing for years, and of doing things (like sliding down a waterslide) you've never dreamed of doing?

Deliver us from feeling insecure and vulnerable.

We much prefer *Armed and Dangerous*.

Daphne's story:

"I get so excited about every pound I lose!"

On a February night during one of the coldest winters in history, Daphne and three friends drove 40 miles to attend one of our seminars. Well, determination like that is sure to pay off. Less than two months later, Daphne wrote us a letter and said:

> To date, I have lost 26 pounds and feel wonderful. People are noticing my weight loss and that really encourages me

to keep it up. My friend and I walk for 45 minutes at least six times a week.

Daphne identified a problem of eating snack foods, even if they're low-fat. It's something we think is worth passing on to you:

> I found I have to stay away from snack foods because it is easy to lose track of a portion and eat the entire bag. If you're hungry, eat a piece of fruit. You are more likely to eat just one apple than twenty-five low-fat chips.
>
> I switched my family, who are big milk drinkers, from 2 percent to 1 percent milk and nobody noticed. And as a former butter lover, I cut that out completely. I even make the boys' lunch sandwiches without butter, and there have been no complaints.

Alicia's Story:

"Wait'll he sees how his shirts have stretched!"

As women, we're usually expected to be giving and sensitive to the needs of those around us. Or at least that's what men keep telling us....

But, whatever the reason, it tends to be true. And you know what? We think we pay for it—with extra weight and poor health.

We've heard women say, "I'd like to cook those foods (or use skim milk, or work out 45 minutes a day), but my husband/boyfriend/son doesn't like it...."

We know you'd never say anything like that, right? But, just in case you would, listen to Alicia, a woman who joined a church-sponsored shopping tour we conducted and immediately changed her buying habits without telling her husband or her teenage children:

> I didn't say anything to my family, except to tell my husband to drink 1 percent instead of 2 percent milk. That was easy. And the only response from the teenagers was to rave about the flavor of the no-fat baked potato chips. By the way, after months of complaining that the laundry had

been shrinking his shirts, my husband came down one morning to tell me now his pants had stretched—and that was only after one week! Just wait till he sees how his shirts have stretched too!

Craig's story:
One more step toward the Major Leagues.

If you're a guy, you would want to be Craig Hawkins. Because if you were Craig Hawkins, you would be seventeen years old; stand 6 feet, 5 inches tall; be heartbreakingly good-looking; and romanced by major U.S. universities who will provide a first-class education if you'll play baseball for their school.

That's Craig Hawkins as we write this book. But that wasn't Craig Hawkins a year ago.

In summer 1995, Craig Hawkins had all the baseball talent he needed . . . and 60 pounds of fat he didn't need. So, when his mother suggested he listen to his favorite aunt Barb, she persuaded Craig that there may be something to eating low-fat foods and following an effective exercise program. (Along with his great looks, first-class mind and athletic skills, Craig has a quality almost unheard-of in seventeen-year-old boys—he listens to his mother.)

Actually, it began when Craig was ill for a week and stayed home to rest. During his illness, he lost his appetite for hot dogs, potato chips and other fast foods. His mother encouraged him to sample yogurt, bagels and cereal—and as long as he was lying around the house, he might as well read fitness magazines and discover how to lose fat and gain muscle. Craig agreed (with a little encouragement from Aunt Barb, of course). So he began eating low-fat foods and reading labels carefully. He also increased his activity routine, doing exercises that made a positive impact on his weight and muscle shape.

In other words, he grew *Armed and Dangerous*.

By the following spring, Craig had lost 60 pounds of fat and gained 10 pounds of muscle. He also proved he had the determination and willpower to make it in the big leagues, and he grew to enjoy the comments of friends (especially girls) who said things like: "Wow—you look great! What are you doing?"

The encouragement was valuable because Craig's friends still choose junk food as their first choice of nourishment. (Boy, a combination of french fries, cheeseburgers and peer pressure can be a killer for anybody!) But Craig sticks to his low-fat diet. Why? Because he feels good about himself and he wants to have the best possible choice of following his dream to become a major-league ball player. His play has improved, his confidence on the field is high, he has more energy than ever, and don't ever pitch him a fastball low and away unless you don't care about seeing the ball again.

'Course, he's still a little shy about some things. Which is why his aunt Barb is telling his story for him.

Denise's story:
A call for help!

Sitting around the swimming pool is fun, but when Denise and her husband installed theirs, the fun led to added fat. The pool wasn't the direct cause, of course—neither were all the days spent eating hamburgers, steaks and ice cream. But together, they all added 50 pounds to Denise's normal 100-pound weight. When she discovered her dress size had skyrocketed from a 3 to an 11, it was time for help, and Denise called us.

> When I left one of Wendy and Barb's seminars, I was on a real "high." I didn't know that so many foods we could eat and enjoy would be low in fat.... or that so many things I was eating, thinking they were low in fat, were definitely *not*!

Unfortunately, Denise's husband didn't share her concern about low-fat products and exercise, and for quite a while he insisted on gnawing on a thick steak and keeping a supply of potato chips and sour cream dip handy. It took a photograph of him in a bathing suit... and a comment that the diving board on their pool literally creaked from his weight... to bring him around. Denise's husband soon lost 80 pounds and feels as good as Denise, and if this all sounds like one of those evangelical cure-'em-with-aprayer shows you see on television Sunday mornings, well, it's not really. Because there was no miracle at work here. It's just the results of some ordinary people who decided they had been victims of excess fat long enough and were now growing *Armed and Dangerous*—all it took was knowledge and determination.

P.S.   *Both Tracy and Denise now work with us, presenting low-fat eating and fitness concepts at our seminars. Come out and meet them sometime!*

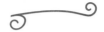

CHAPTER FOURTEEN

Now It's Up to You

If you've read this far, you must be hooked on the idea of reducing the fat in your diet and increasing the level of your physical fitness. We also hope you know that there doesn't have to be a lot of pain or sacrifice involved. In fact, you should be enjoying yourself in almost everything we've talked about until now!

★ You should be enjoying the taste of the foods you eat— to the point (trust us on this, because we keep hearing it over and over again!) where foods that are high in fat are less appealing as time goes by.

★ You should be enjoying the activity you're doing, and actually "listening" to your body as it responds to the new muscle strength you're building.

★ You should be enjoying the comments of friends who notice (and they will!) the improvements in your appearance and attitude.

★ Most of all, you should be enjoying the new feeling you get of confidence in choosing the foods you eat and the way you treat your body.

Do you still feel the way you did?

Remember how we asked if you agreed with some ideas in the early chapters of this book? We also asked you to write reasons why you didn't agree with those ideas.

We did this because many people are skeptical about eating low-fat foods and keeping fit. They tend to be dubious for one (or sometimes both) of these reasons:

1. It doesn't matter what I eat or what I do, I'll always look and feel the way I do today.

2. Even if Wendy and Barb have the solution, I don't have the willpower to make it work.

If you disagreed with any major item at the time, go back now to those notes you made and ask yourself these questions:

★ Do you still feel that way? If not, scratch it out!

★ Do you disagree with a fact or an opinion? We've had every conceivable fact checked by experts—which doesn't mean experts are always correct of course. But before you disregard the facts, please check them yourself. If you disagree with an opinion, that's your right. But we found a way to become stronger both inside and out, and we're spreading the word among others who want to become just as *Armed and Dangerous* as we are—and stay that way.

★ Do you not believe you can achieve all that we did? You may be right—you may also be able to achieve *more* than we did. *Prepare to surprise yourself.* Spend two weeks following our cruise-control formula (eat no food that derives more than 30 percent of its calories from fat) and walking as briskly as you are able for 35 to 40 minutes a day. When the two weeks are up, ask yourself how you feel—and how you look. We don't promise a miracle, but we expect you'll feel and see the difference.

★ Join forces with your partner or a friend. Neither one of us could have accomplished all that we have alone, so why should you be expected to change your life entirely on your own? Talk your spouse into taking part. Or talk your best friend into taking part. If they are one and the same person, aren't you the lucky one? How can they fail to support you?

★ Celebrate everything you achieve! Losing weight and improving your fitness level is a victory worth patting yourself on the back about. Set yourself an affordable award for your achievement—new lingerie or some costume jewelry you've had your eye on.

★ Use every achievement as a stepping-stone to the next one, and the next.

Ten steps to becoming Armed and Dangerous

We've managed to summarize all the basics of *Armed and Dangerous* in ten steps. Follow them one by one, checking off each as it is accomplished. Then start making promises to yourself . . . and keep them!

1. ❑ Let your physician know what you're up to.

We have no doubt that your doctor will wholeheartedly approve your decision to lose weight and improve your overall cardiovascular performance. But let him or her know what you're up to, and have a checkup to identify any physical problems that are likely to arise.

2. ❑ Put your bathroom scale in the closet and leave it there.

Don't even think about losing weight for the first few months. Concentrate on losing body fat. If your physician can provide the data, ask for a measurement of your current body fat when having your physical examination. Have it measured every three months for a year—that's how to plot real progress.

3. ❏ Remember that you have to eat in order to lose weight.

Don't starve your body into thinking there's a famine going on. Plan to eat as much food as you eat now—maybe even more! Just change the *kinds* of foods you eat.

4. ❏ Never let yourself get overhungry.

Denying yourself food is no answer. Eat when you're hungry, and you'll find it easier to maintain your good eating habits. Waiting until you're ravenous means your stomach's desperation may overcome your brain's wisdom.

5. ❏ Balance your fat intake.

We're talking low-fat, not no-fat. We encourage the use of no-fat ingredients but only to balance other foods with higher-than-desired fat levels, such as egg yolks and cooking oil. Use the cruise-control method: Read the labels, measure the fat grams, calculate the calories and divided them by the total. Start by eliminating any food over 30 percent calories from fat, and eventually cut back to 20 or 15 percent.

6. ❏ Remind yourself: It takes both low-fat and activity to grow strong.

Reducing your fat intake will have a positive effect on the way you feel, but it's only one-half of the recipe. The other half is increasing your activity level by elevating your heart rate and maintaining it for a period of time through walking, running, cycling or similar continuous activity. Here's the good news: With less fat in your food and less weight on your body, you'll enjoy the exercise more than you would have in the past.

7. ❏ Turn your fat-storing body into a fat-burning body.

Do you recall that mental picture of the oil tank in your basement overflowing because you weren't burning the fuel fast enough? Use it as an incentive to eliminate all the excess fat you currently carry on your body. By reducing the fat "delivery" and "turning up the heat" through activity, you'll prevent the overflow.

8. ❏ Don't permit yourself to get out of breath.

We're talking exercise here, not exertion. If you become so short of breath when walking or running that you can't talk comfortably, slow down.

9. ❏ Resist manipulation.

The chief advantage of becoming *Armed and Dangerous* is the strength you feel in yourself, both mentally and physically. So now that you're armed with the facts about fat levels in food, you're prepared to resist the manipulations of food advertising—either fast-food items or unhealthy supermarket products. Each time you see or read about a new food or product, calculate the fat content. Then confirm it with a reading of the label or, in the case of fast foods, an inquiry to the franchise holder. Hey, splurge if you want to—just keep your eyes open and your guard up as you go in. It's your body you're defending!

10. ❏ Make only those changes that are realistic for you.

One more time: *Life is unfair,* and it's unfair in many ways. One of them is that nature and genetics give us widely varying body shapes, many of which are difficult to change and rarely in fashion. So, resist the temptation to look like anyone else except a better version of yourself. Instead, set an immediate goal of reducing excess fat and improving your body's efficiency levels. By achieving that, you'll launch an entire chain reaction. You'll look better outside, feel better inside, and be prepared to tackle the next goal—and the one after that—with greater confidence.

A Last Note from Wendy

This is for the people whose interest in eating low-fat foods and becoming fit is driven more by health concerns than any other reason—especially if you suffer from physical problems, as I did.

Modern medicine is perhaps the biggest miracle of our time. When I think of organ transplants in young children and reconstructive surgery to repair the damage of birth defects and accidents, I am stunned by the skill and dedication of so many physicians, surgeons, nurses and researchers. They literally change lives with their fingertips.

But I think every one of them remains impressed by an even bigger miracle—namely, the human body's ability to repair and improve itself if we just provide the right conditions.

As miraculous as modern medicine is, some challenges are still beyond its capabilities. Arthritis, of course, is the one I'm most familiar with. I thank all the medical professionals who helped me in my search for relief from arthritic pain—they were wonderful, and did all they could.

But the rest was up to me. It was up to me to change the kinds of food I was eating, reducing the fat content to a healthy level. It was up to me to strengthen my body so it could deal with the strain of arthritic joints. And it was up to me to replace high levels of medication with natural endorphins that reduced my pain without affecting other parts of my body.

I'm not promising miracles to anyone. Besides, becoming *Armed and Dangerous* isn't a miracle anyway—the results may be miraculous, but they don't happen with a wave of a magic wand. They happen because you want them to.

So I hope you'll use *Armed and Dangerous* the best way possible: To encourage your own miracle—the body you inhabit which, for all of its faults and weaknesses is uniquely yours and the only one you have—to become as strong and as healthy as it possibly can.

Much love,
Wendy

A Last Word from Barb

In some ways, I wish the woman who moped around my house in the weeks after the birth of my baby boy, Jake, were here now. Because then you could see the contrast between us—not just in looks, but in attitude as well.

Wendy and I have achieved so much together, not just as friends but also as business partners. We have our own line of food products, our own business of alerting and educating people like you to the benefits of eating low-fat foods, and now our own book.

When I was too embarrassed to venture outside, I wouldn't have believed all of this could have happened in a million years—yet it's been barely two years! So please don't assume that whatever you want to accomplish is beyond your ability. It's not. You may take longer to get there than some, but so what? The journey is as important as the destination, and slow progress is better than none at all.

And, once again, do it for whatever reasons are important to *you*. If that means being able to buy a size 12 dress again, that's all the reason you need. When you reach that goal, I know you'll be radiant. When you're radiant, you look beautiful. And we all know the world can always use a little more beauty.

One more thing: People who attend our seminars always comment on how much fun Wendy and I seem to have. Darn right we do! Life should be fun. Eating good food should be fun! Improving your fitness level should be fun!

So have fun … and grow more beautiful!

All the best,
Barb

Wendy and Barb's
Armed and Dangerous

Tear-Out
Shopping Guide

Our Own Products

**(Wendy and Barb's —
"You Won't Believe This Is Low Fat!")**

Bakery

- ❏ *Bikini Brownies*
- ❏ *Double-Chocolate Mint Meltaway Cookies*
- ❏ *Banana Blast Muffins*
- ❏ *Cranberry Lemon Zest Muffins*

Deli

- ❏ *Baba Ghanouj*
- ❏ *Hummus*
- ❏ *Bruschetta*

Eggs and Dairy Products

- Egg Beaters
- Egg whites only
- Skim milk
- Chocolate skim milk
- Astro French Vanilla Yogurt
- Astro Banana-Banana Yogurt
- Astro Lemon Yogurt
- Astro No-Fat Sour Cream
- No-Name® Light Sour Cream
- Nu-Tofu cheeses
- President's Choice™ "Too Good To Be True!"™ Fat-Free Plain Yogurt
- P.C. "TGTBT" Fat-Free Chocolate Milk Beverage
- P.C. "TGTBT" Low-Fat Yogurt with 7-Organic Grains
- Silhouette Yogurt
- 1% cottage cheese
- Alpine Lace Lo cheeses

Fish

- Tuna (in water)
- Sole, halibut, haddock, etc. fillets
- Healthy Bake Frozen Fish Products
- Frozen & packaged – No breading Tuna steaks
- Swordfish steaks
- Canned tuna (in water)

Meat and Meat Substitutes

Turkey
- Ground
- Breast
- Smoked Cold Cuts
- Chicken – White meat, no skin
- Turkey scaloppini
- Lean pork loin and tenderloin (in moderation)

- Veal scaloppini (from the leg – in moderation)

Yves Veggie Cuisine Products:
- Hot dogs
- Pepperoni
- Back bacon
- Cold cuts

Condiments, etc.

- ❑ P.C. Appletreet™ Apple blend
- ❑ Ketchup
- ❑ Horseradish
- ❑ Hot sauce
- ❑ Relish
- ❑ Vinegars
- ❑ P.C. Gourmet Barbecue sauce
- ❑ P.C. Jalapeno Jelly
- ❑ P.C. "TGTBT" Natural Pasta Sauce
- ❑ P.C. "TGTBT" Tomato & Vadalia Onion Dressing
- ❑ P.C. Fat-Free Whipped Dressing
- ❑ P.C. Mild White Corn & Black Bean Salsa
- ❑ P.C. Fat-Free Pourable Dressings
- ❑ P.C. Memories of™ Sauces, Dressings and Marinades
- ❑ Healthy Choice Tomato Pasta Sauce
- ❑ Corn syrup/maple syrup
- ❑ Honey
- ❑ Jams and Jellies
- ❑ Golden Dipt Low-Fat Fish Dips
- ❑ Weight Watchers Mayonnaise
- ❑ Kraft Ultra Low-Fat Salad dressings
- ❑ P.C. Fat-Free Mayonnaise

Snacks

- ❑ Fruit
- ❑ Air-puffed popcorn
- ❑ P.C. "TGTBT" Low-Fat Multigrain Pretzels
- ❑ P.C. Low-Fat Chewy Granola Bars
- ❑ P.C. "TGTBT" Low-Fat Potato Chips
- ❑ Frito-Lay Baked Potato Crisps
- ❑ Smart Temptations Tortilla Chips
- ❑ Tostitos Baked Tortilla Chips
- ❑ Mr. Pita Pita Snacks
- ❑ Mr. Pita Bagel Chips
- ❑ Tuffy's Nuts and Bolts
- ❑ No Name Low-Fat Crispy Rice Marshmallow Squares

Bakery Products

- ❑ Angel-food cake
- ❑ Crumpets
- ❑ Pumpernickel bread
- ❑ Sourdough bread
- ❑ Baguettes
- ❑ P.C. Splendido™ Italian-Style Flat Bread
- ❑ Dempster's fruit breads
- ❑ Bagels
- ❑ English muffins
- ❑ Whole-wheat bread
- ❑ Weight Watchers hamburger buns
- ❑ P.C. Greek-Style Pocketless Pita
- ❑ Pita flatbread
- ❑ P.C. Low-Fat Fruit Bars (e.g. Raspberry)

Packaged Foods

❑ Oatmeal
❑ Rice – especially basmati
❑ All cereals under 30 % fat
❑ Primo Bean & Pasta Soups
❑ P.C. "TGTBT" Instant Soup
❑ P.C. "TGTBT" Caribbean-Style
  Jump-Up™ Soup
❑ P.C. "TGTBT" Ready-to-Serve
  20-Bean Soup
❑ P.C. "TGTBT" Pre-Cooked
  Great Northern Beans
❑ P.C. "TGTBT" Pre-Cooked
  7-Bean Mix
❑ P.C. Complete Fajita Package (frozen)

❑ P.C. "TGTBT" Low-Fat Instant
  Black Bean Dip (dry mix)
❑ P.C. "TGTBT" dry soup mixes
❑ P.C. Couscous – plain and whole wheat
❑ P.C. "TGTBT" Mexican-Style One-Step
  Pasta & Beans Radiatore with
  Red and Black Beans
❑ P.C. "TGTBT" Italian-Style One-Step
  Farfalle & Pinto Beans
❑ P.C. "TGTBT" Moroccan-Style One-Step
  Tricolor Coils with Pinto Beans & Lentils
❑ Beans and Peas – dried and canned
❑ Pasta – fresh and dried
❑ Pancake mix
❑ Couscous

Desserts

❑ P.C. "TGTBT" Gelato – Fat-Free, Cholesterol-Free, Frozen Dessert
❑ P.C. Sherbet
❑ Popsicles
❑ Frozen strawberries and raspberries
❑ Haagen-Dazs Frozen Yogurt & Bars
❑ P.C. Light Cheesecake
❑ Snackwell products (Read the labels for under-25 % fat content)

Beverages

❑ P.C. Low-Calorie Fruit Rush™ Drinks (e.g. Peach Melba, Apple Cider)
❑ P.C. Extra-Rich Chocolate Flavor Drink Mix

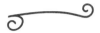

Index